Quinns' Best

By Dick Quinn and Kelly Quinn

A collection of the best from
Help Yourself to Health

Cover Design by Mike Traver
Typography by JEZAC Type & Design
Photography by Doris Doyle, the White Coyote

Quinn's Best

ISBN 0-9632839-4-4 $12.95

**R.F. Quinn Publishing Co.
811 East 48th Street
Minneapolis, MN 55417
1-800-283-3998** (Order Line)

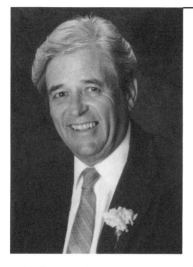

Dick Quinn has been a writer since 1958, but he didn't become interested in health issues until 20 years later.

After a heart attack and failed bypass surgery in 1978, he discovered a common kitchen spice that saved his life. It was Cayenne Red Pepper. He has taken Cayenne every day since to prevent heart attack, control blood pressure and cholesterol, maintain good health and provide energy.

In March, 1992, he published *Left for Dead* which has become a best seller. Mr. Quinn has traveled extensively, telling the *Left for Dead* story on hundreds of radio and TV shows.

Quinns' Best, written with his daughter Kelly, is his second book. He lives in San Clemente, California.

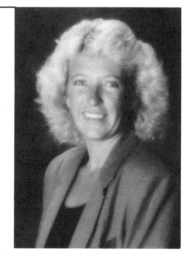

Widowed and diagnosed with chronic hepatitis at age 32, **Kelly Quinn** regained her health through the use of herbs. After much research and experimentation, Kelly was convinced that herbs are a safe, effective alternative to conventional medicine.

An experienced radio announcer and newspaper columnist, she used her new-found energy to spread the word about natural remedies in the publication *Help Yourself to Health*, the audio-cassette *Left for Dead/Remedies* and the book *Quinns' Best* with her father, author Dick Quinn.

Healthier and happier than ever, Kelly has since remarried and lives in Southern California with her husband and their five children where they enjoy experimenting with herbs and helping people help themselves to health.

CONTENTS

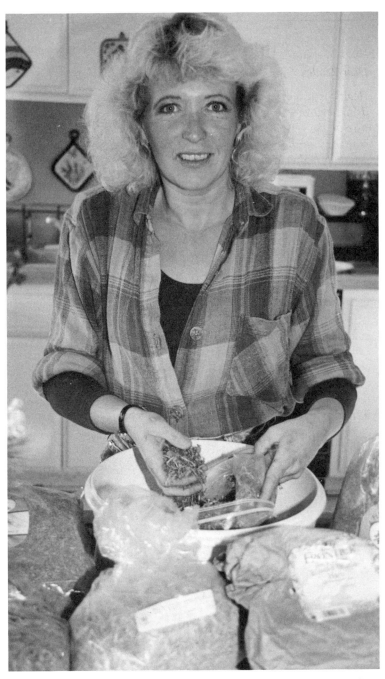

Kelly mixes up a big bag of herbal tea, then brews it by the pitcher.

Dear Reader,

Health is a hot topic these days. We worry about what we eat, drink, smoke, our cholesterol and our stress level. Every time we turn on the TV, pick up the paper or a magazine, we're bombarded with new medical breakthroughs, new rules for longer life, new solutions and new fears. How is anyone supposed to keep up with it all?

That's where we come in. _Help Yourself to Health_ brings you the latest health news in a brief, easy to read and understand format. We want to give you access to information and enable you to make your own healthcare choices. Each of us is a patient at some point in our lives, even if we're simply attempting to prevent illness by eating certain foods.

As patient advocates, we want you to have the information you need to manage your own health. It doesn't matter what you do with the information, but it is important to us that you have it. If you fear getting cancer and decide to increase your intake of beta-carotene rich foods, vitamins C and E, good for you. If you don't care and want to buy a carton of cigarettes, it's your choice. The important thing is that YOU make your own choices. Too often, they are made for you by drug manufacturers, the medical establishment, the FDA or others with something to gain.

We don't have an ax to grind. We accept no advertising or drugs, medicines or medical services. We will tell you the truth. We don't care how bizarre something sounds if it works. We will also tell you if it doesn't and what side effects are involved. After all, as patients, we endure the illnesses and eventually, do the dying. Too many people die prematurely of cancer, heart disease, improperly prescribed or monitored drugs and dangerous diagnostic techniques. _Help Yourself to Health_ hopes to see more people die of old age.

Take care of yourself,

Kelly Quinn

RELIEVING ALLERGY SYMPTOMS WITHOUT DRUGS

By Kelly Quinn

An estimated 50 percent of Americans suffer from allergies and sensitivities. *Sensitivity* is when the body reacts to something in the environment. *Allergies* differ from sensitivities in that antibodies are produced in response to an allergen. Both conditions result in the release of histamines, which can cause hives, rash, wheezing, sneezing and itchy, watery eyes. Sensitivities come and go, however, allergies are permanent.

The first step in obtaining relief is to determine what is causing the reaction. Be aware of when symptoms occur. Is it around dust, cigarette smoke, outside or petting the family cat? The offending substances may be a bit tricky to uncover, requiring a doctor's assistance to determine if an allergy is present.

Once the cause of the problem is identified, consider your course of action. Avoiding the allergens, if at all possible, is the easiest and most effective tactic.

If avoidance is impossible or impractical, desensitization with allergy shots or other treatment can have positive results for some sufferers. Allergy shots consist of a diluted mixture of positive allergens injected into the body, following the theory the body will become used to the allergens after an initial aggravation of symptoms.

A similar method is used with homeopathic allergens, in which a mixture of 6X dilutions are administered 3 times daily. Experience shows desensitization with a marked reduction of symptoms in three to six months.

During desensitization and peak allergy season, sufferers need to control the symptoms without side effects. Stress on the adrenal and immune system also increases the body's requirements of vitamins C, E, B_6, B_5, B_3, and Zinc.

Recent fatal side effects linked to Seldane and Hismanal, antihistamines previously touted because they don't cause drowsiness, illustrate the need for alternative methods of treatment. Fortunately, there are options that are both safe and effective and definitely worth exploring. The following is a partial list of some of the most popular, most of which can be found at your local health food store or co-op.

Freeze dried stinging nettle blocks histamine release. Without histamines, the body avoids the accompanying symptoms of watery eyes, sneezing, running nose and hives. A small percentage of those who take stinging nettle will develop a rash (a possible allergic reaction to the herb itself), but such occurrences are rare.

Anise, a licorice-flavored plant is good for upper respiratory problems, including bronchitis, coughs, and stuffy noses. Modern studies support its effectiveness for those ailments, including relief for asthma sufferers. Two chemicals in the plant: creosol and alpha-pinene, loosen bronchial congestion, making coughs more productive. Hippocrates recommended anise for clearing mucus from air passages. Anise seeds provide the benefits and can be obtained at health food stores and are easy to grow at home. Make a tea with 1 teaspoon crushed seeds to one cup boiling water. Steep 10-20 minutes, drinking three cups daily for maximum effect. Anise can cause minor discomforts like stomach upset or diarrhea, if those appear, discontinue use.

Black mustard alleviates chest congestion in poultices and hot footbaths. The footbaths also banish headaches. For a footbath, add 1 tbsp. dried mustard powder to hot water. For a poultice, try 1 tbsp. mustard to 4 tbsp. flour. Mix ingredients in a bowl with enough warm water to make a thick past. Fold two large white linen cloths (men's handkerchiefs are fine), add paste and apply to chest.

Peppermint and spearmint can be helpful to asthma sufferers. Add essence of mint to 1/2 teacup of warm water. The resulting mixture should be bottled and corked. When there is shortness of breath, a few drops sprinkled on a cloth and inhaled brings relief. It can also be sprinkled on a pillow to be inhaled during sleep.

Slippery elm was used by Native Americans for sore throats, coughs and bronchial congestion. To make a tea, boil from 1-2 tbsp.

of powdered bark to 1 cup water. Drink up to three cups daily.

If you've tried these remedies and have not gotten relief, you may want to try ephedra. It is a powerful bronchial decongestant and not without potentially unpleasant side effects, however, sometimes the symptoms of allergies and colds are so debilitating, it takes something strong to bring relief.

Ephedra's active ingredients are ephedrine, pseudoephrine and norpseudoephrine. These are powerful stimulants which open up bronchial passages to ease breathing. A likely time to try ephedra is when an asthma attack is underway and quite advanced. Pseudoephrine is an active ingredient in many cold and allergy medications today, including Sudafed. Side effects can include increased blood pressure, insomnia, irritability and hyperactivity, particularly when combined with caffeine. A tea brewed from ephedra can alleviate colds, hay fever and asthma.

What do you do if you just don't have the time or desire to make teas and apply poultices? It may not yet be time to rush to the doctor's office for a prescription. Herbal combinations for allergy symptoms are available. The primary ingredient is usually ephedra with a variety of herbs added to address specific complaints. Lobelia is often used to dilate the bronchioles and clear the lungs. Goldenseal is used to repair mucus membranes and marshmallow to soothe, among other herbs.

What happens if you experience an allergy attack and are unable to get to your usual treatment? Find a convenience store or look in the nearest kitchen. Lemonade is a natural decongestant as well as a fine source of vitamin C. Strong coffee can stop an asthma attack and cayenne red pepper added to a little tomato juice or other palatable liquid can help loosen nasal and chest congestion and ease sinus pain and pressure.

What about the allergy-sufferer's lifelong dream to get a pet? Research shows that cats bathed a minimum of once a week will stop producing the dander which causes allergic reactions within three months. Getting Kitty in the bath may be a trifle difficult, but those who have solved their cat-allergy problems by that method claim the younger the cat is, the faster it gets used to bathing.

Similar results have been claimed by those with allergies to dogs. Also, some believe the cause of the reaction is more of a food-sensitivity in the dog and that changing Fido's diet has some beneficial effects. If that doesn't work, consider getting a pure-bred poodle. Poodles rarely cause allergic reactions as the fur on a poodle is almost identical to human hair.

When suffering allergy symptoms, it is important to get relief. It does not do to simply let the symptoms continue unchecked or let it "run its course" as doing so forces the body to deal with the symptoms of allergy as if it were dealing with an illness. This results in a weakening of the immune system, leaving the body open to other illnesses. Congested sinuses can easily become a sinus infection if the congestion is not relieved and the mucus allowed to drain. By the same token, asthma sufferers have more frequent occurrences of bronchitis and pneumonia than those who suffer few attacks. For maximum effectiveness, symptoms should be treated as soon as they occur, rather than waiting for a full-blown allergy attack in which remedies may be of little benefit.

Fortunately, herbal and homeopathic combinations can be very effective in treating the symptoms of allergies. With a program of avoidance, desensitization and symptom control, most allergy sufferers can live virtually symptom-free, without the worry of side effects of conventional treatment.

Can't Sleep? Safe Alternatives to Drugs

By Kelly Quinn

Everyone has occasional times when sleep doesn't come easily. When insomnia becomes chronic, many people head right to the family doctor, where they are given a prescription for tranquilizers. Tranquilizers at best offer only a temporary respite from sleeplessness. The potential side effects, including insomnia, addiction and personality changes can be debilitating and hazardous.

For example, the sleeping pill Halcion has been linked to depression, anxiety, paranoia and violence in some patients. Both Zanax and Valium have been shown to be addictive with long-term use. Another problem with prescription tranquilizers is they do nothing to correct the underlying problems disruptive to a good night's sleep.

Fortunately, there are other ways to combat the problem. One way is to remove sources of stress from the bedroom. Use the bedroom as a place to rest, rather than an office, movie theater or study. Try to ease up on responsibilities. Set aside time before bedtime to wind down from the day.

Limit naps to 20 minutes and don't nap within six hours of bedtime. Avoid alcohol within two hours of bedtime and don't overindulge. Alcohol may make one feel drowsy, but the effects are short-term leading to wakefulness within a few hours after dozing off.

Stay away from caffeinated beverages and avoid heavy meals before bedtime. Exercise more, but not within four hours of bedtime. Physical exhaustion can work wonders in facilitating sleep and exercise reduces stress and tension. Exercise raises the metabolism and the resultant burst of energy will make sleeping difficult if undertaken too close to bedtime.

If a good night's rest is still elusive, there are safe, gentle foods and herbs one can try. L-tryptophan has been used as a sleep aid for many years. However, after a contaminated batch caused fatalities, it has been pulled off the market. L-tryptophan, while no longer available in pill form, is naturally occurring part of many of the foods we eat each day. Ever notice after Thanksgiving dinner how tired and groggy everyone becomes? It's not only due to the large quantity of food consumed, but also due to the high amount of L-tryptophan present in turkey. Milk is another excellent source and gives credence to drinking a glass of milk before bedtime to help one sleep.

Valerian is an excellent sleep aid. While it smells and tastes terrible, it promotes relaxation while countering the effects of insomnia, anxiety and nervousness. Approximately two teaspoons full of powdered valerian to a cup of hot water makes an extremely effective tea. Adding lemon or honey can make the tea more palatable.

It is also available in pill form. A little does the job. Excessive amounts can result in a feeling of grogginess. Cut back as needed.

Chamomile is a marvelous sleep aid. It can be purchased in flower, tea bag, extract or fresh organic form. It is said to be a safe way of assuring even toddlers get a good night's sleep. For tea, add one or two tablespoons of chamomile flowers to a cup of boiling water. Drink half a cupful at a time.

Clove oil is also used as a sleep aid. One can use either whole cloves or clove oil. When using whole cloves, steep them in boiling water, then simmer for several minutes taking care not to let too much water evaporate which could make the resultant tea more potent than required. A teaspoon of clove oil to a cup of hot water will produce a mild, slightly sedative tea. Bruised cloves added to chamomile, linden or peppermint tea can be effective in reversing mild depression.

Hops is a highly effective sedative. Insomnia sufferers should try a wine glass full of hop infusion at bedtime. To prepare, add one ounce hops to one quart water and simmer until about one pint of liquid remains. One can even make a hop pillow to facilitate sleep. Use a muslin pillowcase, slightly smaller than a regular sized case and fill it loosely with dried hops. Attach it to the regular pillow and relax.

Passion Flower is the biggest selling sleep aid in Europe. It is easy to take, just pick up a bottle at your local health food store. It is also a major ingredient in many natural sleep aid formulations on the market and in some teas. Sleepytime tea contains a blend of herbs known for their relaxing qualities.

Keep in mind that people vary in the amount of rest required. Some do well on as little as five hours a night, others swear they need nine or more. Individual needs vary as well. Illness, stress and weather can account for restless nights. Allow yourself some leeway. Sleep deficits can not be corrected in one night, it takes several days. Keep regular hours and remember, simply resting quietly has positive effects.

"We all agree your theory is crazy, but is it crazy enough?"

—Niels Bohr, Nobel Laureate in Physics

Herbal Treatment

FOR THE

Lymphatic System

By Dick Quinn

I am often asked about herbs that might be effective against Hodgkin's Disease and other types of lymphatic cancer. Apparently "orthodox" treatments often cause complications and can't prevent recurrence. In fact, the New England Journal of Medicine for Sept. 21, 1989 says "Secondary cancers are known complications of the chemotherapy and radiation used to treat Hodgkin's Disease." Naturopaths feel that only cleansing and strengthening the body will defeat cancer and other "incurable."

The human body has several systems. Some medical disciplines identify five systems, others as may as nine. Everyone includes the circulatory, respiratory elimination, neurological, digestive and lymphatic or glandular systems. Each system provides something to the whole body and plays a vital role essential to health.

Just as electrical signals move through the neurological system and blood moves through the circulatory system, lymph fluid produced by glands called lymph nodes moves through the lymphatic system, which filters toxins from the blood. Naturopaths feel Hodgkin's Disease and other types of lymphatic cancer are an immune failure caused by toxins in the lymphatic system, which must be cleansed to restore health and prevent recurrence.

Get cleansing started with a one day fast (water only), and two days consuming fresh juice only, followed with a diet of fruit, raw vegetables and raw almonds (10 per meal for protein).

It's vital to circulate the lymph fluid while you cleanse with nutrition and herbs. Just as the heart is the pump for your circulatory system, there are pumps for your lymphatic system. Dr. Carson Pierce, noted cancer specialist, says exercise on a trampoline is the best way to circulate lymphatic fluid. Deep breathing also activates the pumps. If the patient is bedridden, have him lie on his back. Stand at his head and place the heels of your hands just below the collar bone and apply pressure as he exhales at 18 cycles per minute for 10 minutes. Brisk walking also activates the pumps. Whatever pumping method is used, it should be done as often as possible.

The herb called **cleavers** is the ideal cleansing and strengthening tonic for the lymphatic system because it contains needed nutrients and has a detoxifying action. It should be taken as a tea (at least 3 cups per day) and in capsules. Cleavers (also called goosegrass) can be grown as a garden vegetable. Use the dried above ground parts of the plant. The juice is also beneficial.

Echinacea *(ek-in-asia)* **Augustifolia** is the best herb for building the immune system and is commonly used to combat AIDS, leukemia and lymphatic disorders. It stimulates interferon production and dramatically boosts disease-fighting white corpuscles and T-cells, which surround and destroy viral invaders in the blood.

Although some herbalists suggest taking echinacea as a tea, it's very expensive, so you might find it more cost efficient to take it in capsules. Depending upon your condition, take one or two capsules with each cup of cleavers tea, so the herbs combine in your stomach.

There are at least seven different kinds of echinacea, a tall perennial flower you can grow in your garden. Most effective is the root of echinacea augustifolio, which takes four years to develop.

Another powerful anti-microbial herb is **burdock root**—a remarkable effective blood cleanser that is said to kill cancer tumors and a wide range of infections. It's also inexpensive and safe to take with no side effects or overdose danger. Burdock is readily available in capsules and can be drunk as a tea, but it's very bitter.

Goldenseal is yet another anti-microbial herb that prevents and controls infection. It is especially effective when combined with myrrh, which stimulates the production of infection-fighting white blood cells.

Saw palmetto is the herb that provides unique nutrients for the glandular system itself. Herbalists include saw palmetto in a lymphatic formula, because they feel it will take cleansing and healing herbs like echinacea to the glands most efficiently. **Cayenne** is included to promote synergism among the herbs, speed their actions and power the formula.

Many of the herbs recommended here are available in health food stores or can be ordered by them. Some come in pre-mixed combinations; others as individual herbs in capsules or as teas. You might want to do your own combinations by taking capsules of each together or mixing the teas, or you may want to buy your herbs in bulk and mix your own.

TEA FOR THE GLAND

2 parts Cleavers
1 part Burdock
1 part Echinacea (optional, if taken in capsules)
Sweeten with honey.
Optional additional ingredients:
1 part Red Clover
1 part Chaparral Leaves (so effective the FDA will ban it)

Use 1 scant tsp. per cup in boiling water. Allow to cool completely to extract every bit of medicinal value. It can be iced. The best way to make tea is with the herbs "free flowing" in the water, without the constraint of tea bag or tea ball. As the tea cools, the herbs will sink to the bottom of the pot or pitcher. Always use vigorously boiling water, but never boil the herbs-rather, pour the boiling water over them.

Drink 3 or more cups per day; no overdose danger. Herbs are best taken on an empty stomach before eating.

FORMULA FOR GLAND CAPSULES

2 parts Cleavers
2 parts Burdock Root
2 parts Saw Palmetto Berries
2 parts Echinacea Augustifolia
1 part Goldenseal Root
1 part Myrrh (blended separately with Goldenseal)
1 part Cayenne Red Pepper

Buy the herbs ground or grind then in your blender or grinder. Saw Palmetto Berries are very hard to grind. Any of the ingredients can be omitted if necessary, since there are several herbs for the glands and several anti-microbials. Blend them thoroughly and fill gelatin capsules, make "bread capsules" or just eat the powder on salads or in juice.

Take 1/4 to 1/2 teaspoonful of the formula three times a day.

Bulk herbs are sold ground or powdered, others are sold as "C & S" (cut & sifted) or as leaves. Powdered or ground herbs are best for capsules, and can be used for tea. Use less powdered herb than C & S or leaves. Some herbs are certified organic or chemical free, others are wild crafted (uncultivated).

As with vegetables in the market, organic herbs and wild crafted herbs usually cost more than the others.

HEALTH TIPS YOU CAN TRY AT HOME

By Kelly Quinn

There are many things you can do at home with common household products to improve your health and quality of life. Before you dash to the drugstore, give some of these a try:

It's summertime and the living is easy. But you got your first sunburn. If there are no blisters, try making soothing compresses of equal part milk and water. Aloe juice is helpful as well. Beware of thick creams or sticky sprays, they tend to seal the heat into the skin, lengthening recovery time. Applying baby oil right after a shower seals in moisture.

If you must use insect repellents, spray them on the clothing rather than the skin. Citronella-oil candles work as well as chemical yard foggers, yet they are much less toxic.

Stumble into some poison oak or ivy? Try washing the area with a brown soap, which removes oily resins. Frequent tepid water baths cuts down the itching as well as OTC cortisone creams.

Terrified of ticks? Forget the hooey about wearing long pants and socks, unless you want to be a tick collector. Take it from a girl who grew up in Tick Central, the fewer the clothes, the better. That way you can tell when a tick is on you and remove it before it bites.

One bit you anyway? No sweat. Don't yank, spray with hair spray, or rub with rubbing alcohol. Baby oil (suntan oil, vegetable oil, or cooking spray, any oil will do). The idea is to cut off the tick's air so it backs away from the bite. I've heard hot air from a hair dryer works as well, but have never tried it.

Beach fried hair? If swimming in salt water, rinse immediately with fresh water. To avoid the effects of chlorine, rinse hair with water before hitting the pool. The hair absorbs the water, lessening the amount of chlorine to be absorbed. Coating hair with conditioner before swimming helps as well.

Somebody get a cut? Stop bleeding and prevent infection with cayenne. This also, believe it or not, stops the pain! Sugar also prevents infection and promotes healing.

Got a bee sting? Make sure the stinger is out. Then make a paste of baking soda and water. Great for bits that itch too.

Sinus headache? Try massaging area with something cold. I used a chilled bottle of beer last summer and it worked better than Advil!

Breaking in new tennis shoes and got a blister? Leave it alone! Nature uses the blister as a cushion to prevent abrading the skin. If it pops, cover lightly with a Band-Aid.

Love to doze in the sun? Keep naps to 20 minutes. More will make you feel tired.

Kids get swimmer's ear? Prevent them by making sure no water remains in ears. After swimming, instruct child to lay on each side for 5 minutes to ensure drainage. A couple of drops of rubbing alcohol in each ear works as a preventative. Do not put warm oil in the ear , as this could lead to infection.

Chapped lips? Use a sunscreen. Also, drink lots of water, as chapped lips also indicate dehydration.

Someone get car sick easily? Try taking ginger. Benedryl can be helpful as well. Avert problems by having the person sit in the front, no reading in the car and keep the window open. Never travel after a big meal. Saltine crackers can also help.

Sunscreens everywhere, but which to choose? Most people need no more than a 15 SPF, 8 SPF is good also. Higher SPF's can lead to skin allergies. Reapply often, especially if sweating or swimming. Apply before going to the beach to allow the sunscreen to be absorbed by the skin. The colored zinc sunscreens offer total protection and are good for noses and under-eye areas. Desitin diaper-rash medication or it's equivalent is cheaper and works as well, some say better than the high-priced trendy colored kind. Just don't let the kids see the tube if you have adolescents.

Beware of perfume in the sun. It could cause skin irritations and discoloration. Insects will become enamored of you as well.

Jellyfish in your area? To treat stings, rinse with water until stinging stops. We used a beer once, but that didn't seem to work as well as water.

Enjoy your summer!

SUNBURN LEADS ME TO TEA

By Dick Quinn

A few weeks ago, I decided to "get some sun"—something I haven't done in years. When I was a kid, I was in the sun all the time, but the sun was friendlier then. At least, I thought it was.

As I have grown older, I noticed the tan on my arms migrated to form unattractive areas of discoloration. A few years ago, light pink spots appeared on my arms.

When I first noticed the spots, they were faint and painless, so I ignored them—until a couple of weeks ago, when I decided to "get some sun."

After a day or two at the beach, the pale red spots became bright red spots, angrier and seemingly larger than before. I went to a dermatologist who in a three or four minute examination (that'll be $65) concluded it looked like a "classic case of chemical poisoning."

"What drugs do you take?" he demanded.

"None," said I. "I only take herbs." With that bit of heresy the examination ended and I was ushered out with directions to buy an SPF45 sun blocker and come back in three weeks, which won't be happening.

I talked to Dr. Carson Pierce, the naturopath, who advised me to clean my blood and get rid of the toxins in it. I then spoke with Al Watson, who suggested basically the same thing.

Al told me something I guess I never thought about. He said everything we drink must be turned to water by our kidneys. Beer, booze, coffee, wine—just imagine the evil stuff my kidneys have had to handle all these years. It's a wonder they work at all. My kidneys really have it tough. I pour on the poisons, heaping abuse on these poor little guys, never giving them a thought. It's criminal.

Al says all my blood goes through the kidneys, too, and through my liver which filters out the toxins. So my system is loaded with bad stuff from eating, drinking, breathing—living. There's no escaping it.

I decided to clean my blood with herbal tea made, of course, with blood cleaning herbs. So that's what I have been doing for the last three weeks and the results have been terrific.

I drink about three liters of tea every day. There's really no room for anything else, only tea, tea, tea. It tastes terrible and that seems to be an important part of its attraction. I lust after its bitterness. When I get up in the morning, it's right to the refrigerator. I bought a new, larger pitcher at a garage sale, so now I make 3 ½ quarts at a time. My daughters drink it, my friends drink it—I have even talked complete strangers into drinking it and now they can't stop. I talk about it constantly, utterly boring everyone out of his wits. Many people have given in and started drinking it just to shut me up.

I may be hated, but I don't care. I feel great.

Actually Kelly won't drink my tea. "Too bitter," she says. She has her own. Hers is sour, which she contends is better than bitter. But they both do the same thing. They both have worked to fix things we didn't know were broken.

When I began this adventure three weeks ago, I had very painful gout or arthritis in my right foot. It had been there for months and months. Now it's gone and my foot is completely healed.

My teeth had been loose and painful, I couldn't stand cold and they ached. I felt they must be riddled with cavities and abscesses. Now my teeth feel wonderful. I don't know how it can be possible, but the tea fixed them. Really. I'm amazed. I could chew rocks. This stuff is fantastic.

I've lost about 10 or 12 pounds. My skin looks better, my color is better, people tell me I look good—even younger. And my red spots have faded to a less threatening pink and shrunk in size. Now I have reason to hope my arms won't fall off. The only problem is that I can't stop drinking the stuff.

We're still working on the formulas, but I am now drinking a combination of blood cleaners, anti-aging herbs and anti-cancer herbs. Here's something you can try.

Blood Cleansing/Anti Aging Tea

4 parts Gotu Kola
2 parts Chaparral leaves
1 part Red Clover blossoms

1 part Neem leaves or 1 part Burdock root
1 part Violet leaves
Honey, ½ teaspoon ground Stevia, or 1 tsp. Licorice to sweeten
  Put 4 or 5 heaping teaspoons of the herbs into a 2 quart pitcher and cover with boiling water. To sweeten, add honey, ½ teaspoon of Stevia herb or 1 teaspoon of Chinese Licorice. Let it steep until cool, when the herbs settle to the bottom, strain and drink (ice if you like).
  That's my recipe; Kelly's is different, but we're both still molding the clay. I'll let you know how this all comes out.

———————————— ❧ ————————————

FOOD FACTS AND FICTION

By Kelly Quinn

When you're into something, you tend to know a lot about it. Food is one of my hobbies. Not cooking, mind you, eating.
  I like to know what to eat that will make me fat, what will keep me slim, what will give me energy and what will keep me healthy. There's a lot of both information and misinformation out there and finding the truth can be a mind-bending experience. See how much of the following you already knew. You might be surprised, as I was, at how pervasive some of the myths really are.
  You're helping your heart if you buy only foods labeled "no cholesterol." Not true. Even foods with no cholesterol can be loaded with fat. Only animal products contain cholesterol, but foods from plant sources such as potato chips, peanut butter, tofu and vegetable oil are very high in fat. Better to read labels for the fat content of food.
  Avoiding eggs lowers blood cholesterol. Not necessarily so. Although eggs are high in cholesterol, they needn't be eliminated

entirely. It's best to give your overall eating habits an overhaul, cut back on fats from meat and dairy products. Remember when using eggs in recipes the amount of fat is divided among all the servings, contributing only a small amount of fat to the end product. Eggs are a good source of protein and lecithin, among other things.

Carbohydrates make you fat. We used to think so, but research shows it's not the bread, pasta, potatoes, cereal or rice that makes us fat, it's what we put on them. Butter, margarine, creamy sauces and peanut butter are just a few of the high-fat, high calorie toppings that make fat and calories soar. Complex carbohydrates are an important source of energy for the body and can actually promote weight loss and lower cholesterol.

Foods labeled "light" or "lite" are good choices for a weight loss plan. Don't trust in "light" or "lite" labels. Even "low-calorie" is suspect. Remember to ask, lighter than what? Lower-calorie than what? Sometimes by just shaving off a few calories or cutting out a gram of fat, the companies sneak by foods that are still too high in both to be part of a weight loss plan, or even a healthy eating plan. Read the ingredients. Often foods lower in fat will compensate by adding sugar or salt. Always check to see how much fat and calories the item contains. Don't go by the title of the product.

Shellfish are high in cholesterol. Shellfish actually contain less cholesterol than previously thought. As a rule, it's low in total fat and much lower in saturated fat than some meats.

Margarine is less fattening than butter. Most people don't realize they are sacrificing taste for an equal amount of fat when using margarine instead of butter. Both contain the same amount of calories, about 100 per tablespoon. Butter contains cholesterol, but as long as you watch your total fat intake, that's OK. Also, consider using whipped butter. It's cheaper than solid butter because an 8 ounce container lasts as long as a full pound. You also cut both your fat and calorie intake immediately, without sacrificing taste.

Skim milk is a poor source of calcium. The only thing missing from skim milk is the fat. Taste differs, but skim milk actually has more calcium than whole milk.

Vitamins give you energy. Vitamins and minerals enable your body to turn food into energy, but they don't supply energy by themselves. Energy is measured in calories and only carbohydrates, proteins and fat have calories.

If you take vitamins, you don't have to eat a balanced diet. Vitamin/mineral supplements can't duplicate the unique balance of nutritional and non-nutritional components found in food. In fact, some vitamins and minerals need food for them to be recognized and assimilated into the body. The basis for good nutrition must be a healthy diet. The idea is to supplement the diet with vitamins, not supplement the vitamins with diet.

Yogurt is a good source of beneficial bacteria. This is a trick question. The answer is: sometimes. Read the label. Some yogurts are little more than skim milk and gelatin. Others may contain the bacteria, but how much can vary greatly due to pasteurization and heat treating. Always look for yogurt with live cultures and be aware that some believe sweeteners can kill the cultures. Frozen yogurts also vary, but can be a good alternative to ice cream as they are usually lower in fat and a good source of calcium.

Two percent milk is healthful since it's low in fat. Another trick question. Yes and no would be the answer here. Yes, 2% milk is lower in fat than whole milk, but it is not as low as 1%, skim or buttermilk. It's a good choice for kids who do need more fat than adults.

Chicken is lower in fat than red meat. As a rule of thumb, yes, but not always. Some cuts of beef and pork have less fat than dark meat poultry. For low-fat meats, choose packages marked "select." They contain less fat and are better cuts of meat. "Choice" cuts are higher in fat, but by looking carefully and trimming excess fat, you can eat a variety of meats.

A drink with sugar is the best way to boost energy fast. Not true. Though you may feel a bit of a "sugar rush" after drinking sugar-laden beverages, there is a sugar "low" that follows. That's because sugar causes a rush of insulin that can cause blood sugar levels to drop below normal, leaving some people more tired an hour later.

Healthy people never eat dessert. Au contraire! They just know how to choose their treats wisely. Fruit is a great dessert, one you should have every day. Some cookies contain lots of fiber and frozen yogurt supplies calcium. Cheesecake every day probably wouldn't be a good idea, but why not get creative with low-fat foods? Strawberries over angel food cake are delightful and contribute no fat to the diet.

Now, hopefully you know more about the food you eat and how to feel and look even better than you do now. Food can be fun. Necessity is indeed the mother of invention and I thought I'd share a few of my low-fat, high-taste recipes with you. I don't like to mess around with portion sizes. If I want to eat a lot of something, I make it so I can. I'm not into restraint, if you know what I mean. But, I hate to be overweight. Try some of these and see what you think. They are easy, cheap and pretty good, if I do say so myself.

TURKEY STROGANOFF

1 lb. ground turkey or turkey breast
1 can cream of mushroom soup
2 small cans mushrooms or pkg. fresh mushrooms
3/4 to 1 cup no fat plain yogurt
1 onion
Soy sauce.

Brown turkey with chopped onion. Pour off any fat. Add soup, mushrooms (drained), and yogurt. Stir. Add soy sauce to taste. Serve on rice or noodles. Enjoy.

TUNA SALAD

1 can tuna, packed in water
Nonfat plain yogurt
Celery
Onions
Assorted spices: chili powder, pepper, garlic powder, etc.

Drain tuna. In bowl, mix up tuna, celery, onion. Add yogurt to desired spread ability. Add seasonings to taste. Serve on bread or rolls.

LOW FAT LASAGNA

8 oz. pkg. lasagna noodles
Low fat spaghetti sauce, any kind
16 oz. container nonfat cottage cheese
Onion
8 oz. low fat mozzarella cheese
Assorted vegetables: zucchini, broccoli, tomatoes, mushrooms, etc.
    (whatever you have that turns you on).

Cook lasagna noodles. Drain and allow to cool. Cover bottom of baking dish with noodles, using about 1/3. Put assorted chopped vegetables on noodles. Cover vegetables with cottage cheese (thin layer, may season with garlic, onion or parsley), cover cottage cheese with thin layer of sauce. Cover with noodles and repeat until you run out of space or ingredients. Cover all with shredded mozzarella. Cover with foil, heat in 375 degree oven until hot, about 40 minutes. Allow to set up about 20 minutes before serving.

No Meat Chili

Assorted cooked beans (pinto, kidney, black, lentils; canned are fine). About 3 to 4 med. cans full.
Two large cans tomatoes
One med can tomato sauce
Chili powder
Celery
Onions
Corn (optional)
Pepper
Garlic powder or salt
Salt

Rinse and drain beans and dump into Dutch oven. Add tomatoes. Chop celery (use the leaves too) and onion and toss in. Add corn if you have it. Season to taste, heavy on the chili powder and pepper, low on the salt. Cook until vegetables are tender. Chili tastes best the longer it is cooked. Serve on rice with cheese on top, if desired.

Bean Enchiladas

Leftover beans (I used thickened black bean soup once, lentils another time, canned pinto beans another), enough to equal a pound of ground beef.
Pkg. enchilada seasoning
Cheddar cheese
Corn tortillas
Canned enchilada sauce (two small or one large can)

Mix beans and enchilada seasoning according to directions on package. Mix a minimal amount of shredded cheese into the mixture. Spoon a stripe onto corn tortillas, roll up and place them seam side down in pan (cake pans are fine). Fill pan so enchiladas are touching. Pour sauce over enchiladas. Top with grated cheese. Cover with foil and bake at 350 degrees until hot. Be creative, I used cooked rice with the beans once when I was low on beans. Serve with salad and salsa.

As you can see, I'm not too exact with measurements. That's because you should be able to be creative and use whatever you want. Don't be afraid to throw in an unusual vegetable. Consider using nonfat yogurt instead of mayonnaise whenever possible, even nonfat mayo has tons of salt. Use beans instead of meat. It's cheap and better for you. Use leftovers whenever possible. Enjoy!

June 1993

Dear Reader,

Things have been hopping here at <u>Help Yourself to Health</u>.

We're working on new ideas, experimenting on ourselves and anyone we can find with an open mind. In February, I put my kids on homeopathic remedies. My son seemed to be on the verge of bronchitis, so I got a bottle of pills for bronchial cough, another for hay fever. I couldn't believe anything so tiny could do so much. I had to chase him down for a couple days as the dose was every two hours during acute attacks. You know what: it worked! No cough syrup was as effective.

Better yet, I wasn't merely suppressing a symptom, he was cured! There were no side-effects and it was much cheaper than a prescription. I made sure he got extra C and drank three dragon cocktails a day (cayenne and tomato juice) as well. I also dabbled in aromatherapy, using a candle for congestion while he slept. It helped some, but nothing really knocked the infection out until I tried the homeopathic pills.

I'm going to continue to experiment. I have a candle for "slimming" and need to drop a few pounds. I'll let you know how it works.

Take care of yourself,

Kelly Quinn

ℋeat Units Tell You Much About Cayenne

By Dick Quinn

ayenne and all other hot food gets its heat from a substance called capsaicin. Some years ago, a man named Scoville developed a means of measuring the capsaicin in food by calculating the food's bite. He called the measurement standard Heat Units Scoville (h.u.s. or simply h.u.). Today, it is the accepted standard for all Cayenne and other hot foods.

Heat units are a unique standard, not to be confused with British thermal units. The number of heat units in Cayenne tells you the amount of capsaicin, which provides the power or energy, so it's a very important measurement. The best parallel is with liquor. 100 proof liquor is twice as strong as 50 proof because it has twice the alcohol and twice the effect. 100,000 heat unit Cayenne is two and a half times as strong as 40,000 heat unit Cayenne, so it, too, has much greater effect. Most people get the energy they need by taking about half as much 100,000 h.u. as they would 40,000 h.u.

The Scoville method of measurement involves a panel of tasters employed by the Cayenne importer (called a "manufacturer"). The Cayenne is soaked in alcohol to make a tincture, then each taster puts a drop on the back of the throat and estimates its heat, according to how much water must be drunk and time pass to kill the burn. The shipment of Cayenne is then assigned a heat unit rating.

It's all so unscientific, it can't possibly work—but it does. In recent years, a machine has been devised that tests heat unit ratings, which has reaffirmed the accuracy of the human testing panel.

Heat unit ratings range from Paprika (a type of Cayenne) at 1 h.u.

to Cayenne oil at 1 million h.u. Nearly all Cayenne at the health store is 40,000 h.u., unless the label says otherwise. Bulk Cayenne from East India ranges from 60,000 to 80,000 h.u., West African Cayenne comes in at 135,000-175,000 h.u. and Habaneros from New Mexico have 275,000-300,000 h.u. Culinary Cayenne from the grocery store has as little as 2,000 h.u. and often has been irradiated.

Capsaicin is in all hot food, but only Cayenne has all five types of capsaicin, so it's most medicinally effective. It is also the only herb with an internationally accepted standard for potency. Cayenne is a capsicum, like a tomato. Both are fruits, not vegetables like jalapenos and other true peppers.

Ginger is often used in formulas to buffer very hot Cayenne and speed its action.

Cayenne can be taken in gelatin capsules, mixed into cold juice or rolled up in bread like a little burrito. Always take it with a cold drink just before eating.

---

*H*ELP *Y*OURSELF *E*ND *B*AD *H*AIR *D*AYS

By Kelly Quinn

*Y*ou thought you could sneak by one more day without washing your hair, but you were wrong. Your clothes look great, everything else is in place and all you can think about is how crummy your hair looks. It's a bad hair day.

We've all had them. Hair is much more than nature's way of keeping our heads warm, hair makes a statement. Only sometimes it says things we didn't want it to. The condition of our hair gives clues to our health and lifestyle. The style we choose expresses who we are and influences how others view us. When our hair looks good, it's easier to feel good.

Considering how much time and money we invest in our hair, surprisingly few of us are completely satisfied with it. We peruse the latest styles in magazines, go to expensive hair stylists, keep a ready stock of shampoos and conditioners and buy any number of bizarre products, all in the quest for the perfect head of hair.

We're easy marks for any charlatan who'll promise us a thick, shiny mane. Look at the ingredients in your shampoo. Does it contain formaldehyde? That's a known carcinogen. Does your hair dye contain coal tar? That's another. Most shampoos are toxic to children if ingested. Those that smell fruity or like bubble gum are particularly appealing to the little ones.

Ever wonder how products deliver on their promises? Remember Protein 21? That was a popular shampoo in the '70's which promised to mend split ends, a big problem for those of us who wore our hair long. You can still get it in Mexico, but I haven't seen it here in years. My uncle compared its ingredients with those in glue, and they were similar. If all it took was glue to fix our split ends, wouldn't a giant economy size of Elmer's have been cheaper?

Hair dryers, curling wands, perms, coloring and hot rollers damage hair. Shampoos, conditioners, mousse, gels and sprays leave our hair dull and lifeless. So we dash right out to buy more.

Or we give up. Maybe you put off washing your hair because the constant disappointment finally got to you. Not to worry, try a dry shampoo. **Talcum powder, cornstarch, oatmeal, cornmeal** and **bran** work well. Just sprinkle about 2 tablespoons on your head, keeping it near the roots. Leave on for about three minutes and brush out. Excess oil is absorbed and hair has a new lease on life for the day. I've tried this and it's a lifesaver!

The time has come to have the hair you've always dreamed of. Read on for recipes for conditioners that will nourish the hair without coating it, tips for styling and protecting your hair, rinses that will add color safely¡even things to try if you fear losing your hair. All that you can do at home without spending a fortune or taking a course in chemistry.

For example, what do you do if you're in a place without water, but your hair needs freshening? Maybe you're camping and have nothing of powdery consistency to absorb the oils and dirt. Try this:

Find a couple of **eggs**. Whip the **whites** to a frothy consistency and apply to hair. Allow to dry, then brush out completely.

You've overdone the conditioner and your hair just lays there like a dead animal. Just hang your head upside down and spray a tad of **hair spray** underneath. Use any kind or make your own.

HAIR SPRAY FOR FINE HAIR

1 lemon
2 cups water

Chop lemon. Add lemon to water in top of a double boiler. Simmer until liquid has been reduced by one-half. Strain through cheesecloth and pour into a clean pump-spray bottle. Add ½ cup water to thin mixture if necessary. Keep refrigerated. Make a new batch every few days as this contains no preservatives. For **dry hair** substitute an **orange** for the lemon.

Not into hair spray? No problem. For the '90's look, try a **beer mousse**. Use one half can of beer and work it through the hair. Style as usual. As the beer dries, the smell disappears.

Avoid the problems of over conditioning and styling product build-up by deep-cleaning hair every other week or so. Add two tablespoons of **baking soda** to your favorite shampoo. Wash hair, rinse and apply conditioner. If your hair is permed or color treated, you may want to spot-test an area first.

It's Friday night and while you look great, your hair looks like you just stuck your finger in an electrical socket. It's dry, frizzy and feels like straw. Conditioner doesn't seem to help. Sounds like you need to bring on a deep-conditioning treatment. If you normally have dry hair, you can use **mayonnaise** to deep condition fried ends. Just work the mayo through, avoiding any contact with the scalp. Let it sit for at least five minutes and wash out. Use this treatment before you wash your hair.

Be careful, though, not to use this on hair that tends to be oily. I tried this back in the '70's, but I made a few mistakes. Mistake number 1: I got it on the roots of my hair, though I have naturally oily hair. Mistake number 2: I assumed Miracle Whip was the same as mayonnaise. It's not. I had to wash my hair for hours to get the oil out. Yes, my hair was the softest thing I'd ever touched, but it looked so greasy I didn't want to touch it. So, I know it does work, just keep it away from your scalp.

Another great treatment for dry, damaged hair is **olive oil**. Follow the directions for mayonnaise. **Almond oil** is also good. Or if you're feeling creative, mix one cup **olive oil, one egg** and one cup **honey.** Comb through dry hair and leave it on for three hours. Wash out.

To keep hair healthy, make your own **protein shampoo** by adding an **egg** to a bottle of any kind of shampoo.

If you live next to an ocean, try bathing your head with **sea water** and **seaweed** to condition the scalp.

Summer can be tough on hair. Sunlight, salt water, chlorine and even sweat can fry your hair. To minimize damage from swimming, **rinse** your hair before going in the water. Just use regular water. You can even coat hair with **conditioner** before swimming. The idea is that hair can only absorb so much water, so let it absorb water that won't damage it. Be sure to rinse hair as soon as possible afterwards. Be wary of chlorinated water as it can give blonde hair a green tinge.

To speed lightening from the sun, put **lemon juice** on your hair before hitting the beach. If you don't want the sun to lighten your hair, coat it with **olive oil** mixed with **sunscreen.** Bonus: the oil will condition your hair while you play.

To keep hair color looking it's best, rinse hair with **chamomile tea** or **lemon juice** for blondes. Brunettes use **coffee, tea, red cider vinegar,** or a tea of **walnut leaves.** Redheads use **beetroot juice** or **red cider vinegar.** Rinse out after five minutes.

Here are a couple of rinses you can make at home:

Herbal Rinse for Light Colored Hair

1 cup marigold flowers
1 cup chamomile flowers
½ cup orange peel
½ cup lemon peel
½ cup comfrey root
1 qts. apple cider vinegar

Place herbs in a wide-mouthed container. Pour hot vinegar over herbs. Cap container. Shake well and allow to sit for 10 days, shaking daily. After 10 days, strain herbs through cheesecloth, pressing herbs to extract vinegar. Add two tablespoons to each cup warm water to make rinse. Follow with clean water rinse.

Herbal Hair Rinse for All Types of Hair

½ cup rosemary
½ cup red clover

½ cup nettle
½ cup sage (for dark hair)
OR
½ cup chamomile (for light hair)
½ cup witch hazel leaf or bark (for oily hair)
OR
½ cup marigold (for dry hair)

Mix and store in a covered, light-proof container. To prepare for use: Take ¼ to ½ cup herb-mixture and add to 2 cups water in pot. Cover, bring to slow boil, simmer a few minutes and remove from heat.

After shampooing hair, strain herbs from pot and add cool water to liquid until the temperature is comfortable to your scalp. Pour over hair. Catch drippings from rinse in pot and re-use until gone. No need to re-rinse.

Dry herb mixture makes enough for 4 to 8 rinses.

Now you've got some ideas to improve both the look and color of your hair. Have fun experimenting.

May all your hair days be good ones.

———————————————— ?● ————————————————

*D*ESPERATION *L*EADS TO *T*EA

By Kelly Quinn

I was a basket-case. After a year of struggling with hepatitis, nearly continual pelvic pain and stress, I looked like I may have won the battle, but lost the war.

I looked old. No one would have believed I was only 33. My face was lined, haggard and sagging. To look at me was to see the face of stress.

I felt hideous. I had acne which had started last summer when my husband died and I got sick, but which nothing could alleviate. And believe me, I tried everything. I spent money I didn't have on high-tech creams, blemish and oil control medications and washed my face constantly. I had to, within an hour after cleansing, my face looked and felt oily. I produced enough oil to power the western world.

Plus, if that weren't enough, I always felt tired. I felt I could sleep for a week and not get enough rest. I had no energy, but I forced myself to carry on. I'd gained weight, but no matter what I did, it seemed to stay with me. My liver problems and gynecological disorders made me retain water. Prescription medicine only worked for a couple of days and had negative side-effects. Herbs helped, but I was so tired of having to take pills all day. I'd forget and almost never keep the dose up enough to do me much good.

I was also constantly running from depression. The worst thing for me was to have time to myself, because I'd quickly become overwhelmed with the feeling that life was hell.

So I plodded along, fantasizing about feeling better someday, seeing the memory of who I'd been a year ago quickly fade away.

One day I accompanied my father to a dermatologist. I'd toyed with the idea of making an appointment for my face, but knew any drugs they'd give me would be too hard on my liver. My dad had little red spots on his arms, he looked like he'd been splashed with hot grease or something, but he said it was from going in the sun. Apparently, he'd had them for years and upon exposure to sunlight they quickly got worse. He was concerned it might be skin cancer.

Sure that the appointment would take at least 20 minutes, I wandered around town, stopping in the drug store to see what new concoction I could put on my face. Nothing I hadn't already tried without results.

I went back to meet him and he was gone. I found him having a cup of coffee outside a place we frequent. His appointment had taken less then ten minutes. The dermatologist had told him he had some sort of poisoning, and wanted to know what drugs my dad was taking.

When Dad told him all he takes are herbs, the doctor became hostile. Nevertheless, he didn't think it was cancer, although he made sure to tell Dad he couldn't tell for sure, but that if Dad wore sunblock for a couple of weeks, the spots should be gone. He wanted to see Dad in a couple of weeks.

Dad didn't want to see him again, ever. So, while he was waiting for me, he was planning his next move. He figured if his body was filled with toxins, he'd have to go on a detoxing regimen. He would use blood cleansing herbs and make a tea, and cut out meats, sugar, alcohol and anything that could be harmful.

I didn't see Dad for a couple of days. He had gotten advice from people supporting his theory. He wore his sunblock and every day had a banana with flax-seed oil mixed with onion and a half a walnut. Not a whole one, not two, one half a walnut. And he drank his herb tea. Gallons of it.

When I saw him, I was amazed. He looked fabulous! His skin looked clear and youthful, his color was great and he'd appeared to have lost some weight. I didn't care what his tea was like, I knew I had to have it.

So I took a swig. Immediately, I was hit with the most bitter taste I've ever known. It was like battery acid. On the heels of which was a cloying, overwhelming sweetness. Ugh. I couldn't do it.

I was bereft. I couldn't gag his tea down and it looked like just what I needed.

Fortunately, Dad had the idea that we come up with a tea I could stomach. Only a few of the herbs he uses are bitter. He actually likes the taste of his tea. He also adds stevia, an herb that is a natural sweetener. I, on the other hand, never put sweetener in my tea or coffee.

I went home with a sack of herbs and immediately brewed myself up a pitcher of tea. I used a tea ball for the first batch, but quickly discarded it as it seemed too small for the amount of herbs I wanted.

My tea was better. I drank it, not enjoying it, but I drank it. I didn't notice much, but since I didn't know what else to do, I kept chugging. I found I drank a little more than two quarts a day.

During the first week on the tea, I found some lemons in the bottom of my refrigerator. I chopped them up and threw them in, rind, seeds and all. When my tea was chilled, I had a glass¡it was great! The answer I'd been seeking. It was refreshing and simply delightful. I found myself actually craving my tea.

About the fourth day on the tea, I was out for my morning walk with the dog. I'd stopped working out a few weeks earlier, I just didn't seem to have any energy or enthusiasm for it. Usually, I'd trudge home and collapse, completely wiped. That day, however, I was › of the way home when I realized¡I felt great. In fact, I wanted to exercise. I got home and pulled out my stairmaster. I'd retired it months ago when the cable broke, but had recently repaired it, fantasizing I'd use it again someday.

I dragged it in from the garage, leaped on and started working out. It felt great! After about five minutes, the cable snapped again and rather then feeling relieved, I was frustrated. So, I dragged out my step platform and worked out on that. Afterwards, I was drenched with sweat, but I felt wonderful!

I started wearing wrist weights when I went for walks. It felt great to work my muscles. I realized I hadn't felt this good since last year.

And, my face started clearing up. Usually, I'd get out of the shower and a sunbeam would hit me, showing my awesome case of acne in all it's splendor, sending me into major depression. I mean, how do you hide your face? Veils just aren't in fashion in this country. Every time I'd get close enough to someone to speak to them, I'd be sure they were looking in awe and revulsion at my face. Now, a couple weeks after drinking the tea, my face looked smoother, with very few breakouts.

I knew the real test would come just before I got my period. I usually suffered major breakouts, headaches, pelvic pain, bloating and was ravenously hungry, the seven days preceding the onset of my period. Since I always seemed to be either going into another cycle, or just coming out of one, I didn't bother to keep track of when to expect it. I usually knew it was coming weeks in advance.

Imagine my surprise one day when it came and I wasn't prepared. That had never happened to me. Thinking back, I realized I hadn't had any major pelvic pain either. The only time I'd been that pain-free was when I was pregnant (which might explain my three kids).

My dad had gone on a three week business trip right before I started on the tea. When he returned, he commented on how much younger I looked. I was pleased, but skeptical. He hadn't seen me in three weeks, maybe he was just glad to see me. Then I saw a friend I hadn't seen in a couple of weeks. She commented on the same thing. So did a neighbor. An acquaintance, talking about her need for a diet, asked how I kept in such great shape! Maybe, I thought, this stuff works after all!

It's like a new life. Sure, things that stressed me out are still there, but I realized I haven't felt despondent since I started the tea. I have minor breakouts on my face when it's hot, but nothing I can't control. I haven't had to spend evenings curled up with my heating pad, or wolfing down pain-killers. I still hold water when it's hot, but not to the extreme I did before.

I was getting my car fixed last week and the receptionist asked me what I was drinking. I told her a little about my tea and she was amazed I'd ever had a major acne problem. I tell you, this stuff is incredible! And it's so easy. I just throw about 2/3 cup of my herb mixture into a pitcher, add boiling water and forget about it. When it cools, I put it in the refrigerator. I fill my water bottle with it and carry it everywhere. In fact, if I'm running low on tea, I feel anxious. I hate wanting a swig of tea and finding I'm out. I used to drink a lot of water, but there's water in the tea. I occasionally have a cup of coffee, but it's a treat. I don't want pop, I want my tea!

I'm going to put my kids on it this week. They are entering the teenage years and complain about their skin and experience the usual teenage mood swings. If it works for me, it should be just the ticket for them. I'll let you know how it works. In the meantime, in case you wanted to try it, here's my recipe for tea. It has changed a few times and I'm still experimenting, but the basic components are all here:

KELLY'S TEA

3 parts Gotu Kola (*Stimulates central nervous system, aids in elimination of excess fluids, decreases fatigue and depression. Good for sore throats, hepatitis, stress, liver and heart.*)

2 parts Chickweed (*Reduces mucus in lungs. Good for asthma. High in vitamin C. Good for gastrointestinal disorders and colds; tumors, cancer skin diseases, acne, appetite suppressant, mild diuretic.*)

2 parts Red clover (*Appetite suppressant, blood purifier, good for skin.*)

2 parts Red Raspberry (*Good for cramps, uterine and intestinal spasms, healthy nails, bones, teeth and skin.*)

½ part Squawvine (*Good for uterine problems, diuretic.*)

½ part Cleavers (*Good for skin, lymphatic system, swollen glands, ulcers and tumors. Diuretic.*)

A "part" can be any measurement, as long as it is consistent. You can use a teaspoon, a cup, whatever. I put 2/3 cup in for 2 quarts. This tea tastes best chilled, but can be drank any way. Try adding lemon juice if you're inclined, I like it that way.

FACE SAVERS
THAT HELP YOU
SAVE MONEY, TOO!

By Kelly Quinn

For the first time in years, I went cosmetic shopping. I was amazed at how much things cost and how much there was to choose from. How many times have you purchased a product and discovered upon returning home that it is not what you thought it was? There are ways to cut the risk of buying the wrong product, the easiest of which is to cut down on what you need to buy.

The reason it had been years since I've bought cosmetics is because I take advantage of the free samples at department stores. If you can find a product you like, wait until they offer a free gift with purchase. Back in the '70's I discovered Estee Lauder's Milk Cleansing Grains and White Linen Cologne. Both easily last me six months at a time. I wait until I'm running low and then start watching the ads in the paper. I've been able to keep my stock of sun products, make-up and even cosmetic bags full ever since. It's a great way to try high-quality, expensive products for free! I need the cleanser or cologne anyway, why not replenish my make-up supply at the same time?

To take advantage of the personnel at the cosmetic counters in department stores. They are usually much better trained than the teenager at the drugstore and can give you tips of what ingredients to stay away from, what shades look best with your complexion, etc. They are usually more than happy to give you pointers and let you try out the products. Just decide in advance that it is a seek and explore mission and that you won't buy anything that day.

From chatting at the cosmetic counter, I discovered the color of blush I'd used for years was the wrong one. I learned to stay away from products containing mineral oil as it would exacerbate my oily skin. And, if you do purchase something, most cosmetic departments will let you return it if you don't like it. How many drugstores will do the same?

The key is to make those purchases count. I've got baskets full of cosmetics and skin creams I never use because I found a way to make better ones at home.

Do you spend a fortune on cleansers? Soap and water may be old-fashioned, but it is also the best. For correcting skin problems, try some of these:

Carrot Cleanser: Cook two carrots until soft, then mash. After cooking, apply the pulp to your face. Let it harden for a few minutes before rinsing. High in Vitamin A.

Nature's Face-lift: Apply beaten egg white to the skin. Let dry then rinse.

Need a Scrub?: Make your own with ground cornmeal and oatmeal.

Smooth and Soften Skin: Make a paste of minced, raw beets and heavy cream. Apply to face, wait 20 minutes, then rinse with cool water.

Spot Repair: Shrink a blemish by holding an ice cube to the affected area for about three seconds. Remove for three seconds, then repeat process twice more. Reduces swelling and redness.

Instant Mask: Use a liquid Pepto-Bismal like product (there are cheap copy-cat versions at drug stores). Cover the face with it, but avoid the eye area. Let it dry, then rinse with cool water.

Save the Skin Around Your Eyes: Break open a vitamin E capsule and spread the oil around your eyes. Better than store-bought eye creams. Good for abrasions, too.

Puffy Eyes?: Potato slices absorb excess water and help eliminate puffiness. Also try sliced cucumbers, cool tea bags.

Moisturizer: Mix non-fat milk with water and spray it on face. Wipe off excess. Yogurt too! Pat yogurt on face. Leave it on for 30 minutes then rinse.

Try and Apple Facial: Peel, cook and mash one apple. Mix it with milk. Let cool, apply to face. Leave on 15 minutes, then rinse.

Try Making Your Own Powder: For face powder, use a dry skillet to brown oat flour, cornstarch, rice flour or white clay until it reaches the desired shade. Store in a tightly covered jar. Apply with a cotton ball.

Body Powder: Forget the pricey, perfumed kinds. Just use cornstarch. For a more upscale powder, buy el cheapo baby powder with cornstarch at the drug store.

Make Sure You Always Have: Petroleum jelly and witch hazel on hand. Petroleum jelly is a fabulous moisturizer for super-dry skin. Works great on elbows, feet and lips too. Witch hazel can even be used as a mouthwash: mix 15 tbs. water and 3 tbs. witch hazel with a few sprigs of mint or lots of lemon peel. It's also a fabulous cleanser. Just use a cotton ball soaked in it.

Home-made Skin Tonic: Extract the juice of two avocados, mix with the juice of one small lemon. Shake well before using.

Flour Cleanser: Wash your face and neck. Mix 2 tbs. flour and 2 tbs. honey with 2 tbs. milk until smooth. Cover face and neck with the paste. Leave on 30 minutes. Rinse and pat dry.

As you can see, with a little time and even less money, you can look fabulous. Isn't it fun to outwit the system? Which leads to the best beauty hint of all: nothing makes a person look better than a smile.

June 1993

Dear Reader,

Summer brings a lot of wonderful memories. When I was a kid in Faribault, Minnesota, we spent summers at a place called French Lake. My father had bought some property on the lake during the Depression, when it was cheap. Everything was cheap then for those who had money to buy it.

The cottage was rather remote in those days. We owned one-half mile of shoreline adjoining more empty shoreline. It was a half mile walk to reach other cottages and the little resort. Now there are cottages everywhere.

I spent most of my time in the water, so I never learned to play baseball like the kids who lived in town, but I sure could swim.

It was the 1940's. Radio was big. I listened to Jack Armstrong every day at 5. Terry and the Pirates was on at 5:30, the Lone Ranger at 6, Captain Midnight at 6:30. At night it was Gang Busters, Fred Allen, and the really scary programs like Inner Sanctum and Lights Out. Radio was so real. Television just can't compare.

The War overshadowed everything. We were all in it together. Hitler and Tojo were the bad guys. Drugs were something you got at the drug store. Guns were used for hunting. Food was safe to eat.

You could trust the doctor. Even the sun was friendly. It really was a "kinder, gentler" time.

One day I was swimming at the resort when my mom and dad came by in our big Plymouth 4 door sedan with the red leather upholstery. I still remember how that car smelled. They were going to a movie in town, the babysitter was at the cottage and would I be all right. I assured them I would. I must have been 7 or 8 at the time.

"Don't drown, honey," my mother said in parting. I remember it so clearly. "Don't worry, mom, I won't drown."

A few minutes later, I was back in the lake swimming out to the diving tower. I could only do the dog paddle, a slow, tiring stroke, and the tower was my absolute long distance limit. When I got there I was always exhausted, so I would grab a bolt or barrel and hold on until I had rested enough to swim around to the ladder on the other side.

That time, I got to the tower utterly exhausted and grabbed for a bolt, but my hand slipped off and I sank, too tired to keep myself afloat.

"Don't drown," my mother had said. I couldn't do that—I had promised I wouldn't—yet I was sinking in deep water, too tired to save myself. I thought about my promise to her as I sank. I remembered the mud at the bottom was icy cold.

Then I realized I didn't have to drown. I wasn't tired any more. I was strong enough to swim again because I had relaxed while I was sinking, rather than fighting to swim and drowning. I had regained my strength in those few seconds, thanks to what my mother had said to me. "Don't drown," she said. So I didn't. Maybe it would be a good thing to tell your kids.

Take care of yourself,

More Help for Bad Hair Days

By Kelly Quinn

Sometimes your hair needs more help than a new conditioner or shampoo. What if you are suffering from **dandruff**; **gray, discolored hair**; or horror of horrors; **hair loss?**

After all, there are many concerns you might have with your hair besides a desire for nice highlights. Take dandruff for example.

Your hair can look utterly fabulous, but you dare not wear dark colors because of flakes that accumulate during the day. Before trading your dark attire for white, take a moment to ask yourself: have I been doing anything unusual to my hair lately?

DANDRUFF

Dandruff can have many causes. Washing your hair too often can dry the scalp. Commercially available hair dyes can damage the scalp, killing skin which later flakes off. I had that problem when using a product that claimed the "most dramatic blonde in one easy step." It blonded my hair, all right, but while I was using it the chemicals burned my scalp.

The next day as I was combing my newly blonde locks, I noticed patches of skin coming off my head. The more I brushed, the more there were. Most commercially available dyes suggest users do a patch test first, but I have yet to meet anyone who really does a test before coloring their hair. Never use dye if you have any irritations or abrasions on your scalp.

I've also been advised to put plastic over my head to "bake" the dye in. Bad idea. While it does seem to make the color really "take," your head can't breathe and damage from the chemicals will be intensified.

In the '70's there was a big to-do about coal tar, a known carcinogen which was in may hair-dyes. I don't know if it's still an ingredient, but do you really want to put something on your head that comes with warnings to stay away from flames, not inhale the fumes and not leave on longer than directed? Hair dye still sounds pretty toxic to me.

What we put on our scalps is indeed absorbed by the body. You probably know that farmers and farm workers have high rates of cancer. But did you know they absorb chemicals through their heads because of the hats they wear? The hat becomes saturated with toxins and while their clothing is washed, hats usually are not. Think about that when you put something on your head. What we apply outside usually finds it's way inside.

Maybe you haven't colored your hair. Have you had a perm? **Permanent wave solutions** can really burn your scalp. No perms either? Maybe it's from **heat styling**. Blow dryers and hot curlers can fry your scalp while they style your hair. Try the old-fashioned way: **air dry** your hair or use **rollers**. The sponge-kind work best and come in an assortment of sizes. You can also roll your hair in **rags** for a tight, perm-style curl. **Hair tape** is another option. Just tape your hair the way you want it to be and allow it to air dry. Don't forget the trick of **braiding** wet hair until dry. You'll look like you had a perm.

Let's say you never style your hair and you still have dandruff. Try a different **shampoo**. You could have a **shampoo build-up** or be using the wrong type for your hair type. Also consider changing **conditioners**. Dandruff is often just dry skin. When you shampoo, use a gentle type and condition scalp well. Just be sure to **rinse well** and **massage** your head vigorously to remove dead skin.

Dandruff can be a result of **stress**. Try to mellow-out by adding exercise to your routine. Follow the above suggestions for gentle treatment of the scalp and see what happens.

You can also try using a **vinegar rinse**. Not only will vinegar remove shampoo build-up, it will often completely eliminate dandruff on the first try. Mix a little vinegar with water or use it straight.

Try putting 30 **aspirins** into a bottle of your favorite shampoo. Let them dissolve and shake well. Use like regular shampoo.

Old-fashioned **tar** shampoos work. Or, if you feel particularly creative, try one of these:

Easy Herbal Dandruff Shampoo

4 tbs. dried thyme
2 glasses water
   Boil thyme for 10 minutes in the water. Strain and allow to cool,

before massaging into clean, damp hair. Leave on for one hour, then rinse in hot water.

Almost as Easy Natural Dandruff Shampoo

Two eggs yolks
½ cup water
Apple cider vinegar
Water
    Beat egg yolks in half-cup water. Massage into hair and scalp for 5 to 10 minutes. Rinse well with water, then rinse again with a mixture of 2 tbs. apple vinegar and water.

Really Creative Anti-Dandruff Rinse

1 cup Witch Hazel Extract
Comfrey Root
Rosemary
Nettle
Lavender
    Add a pinch each of comfrey root, rosemary, nettle and lavender to Witch Hazel Extract. Let steep for 3 to 5 days, until the witch hazel smells better. Strain out the herbs. Apply liquid directly to scalp before bedtime. Sleep. Also makes a great deodorant!

You can also make a tea with any or all of the following herbs: white willowbark, birch bark, chaparral, peppermint, nettle, artichoke leaves, creosote bush leaves, quassia chips, or comfrey root or leaves. Allow tea to cool and apply to scalp. Leave on 10 minutes or so, then rinse with cool water.
    Sunlight is also a treatment for dandruff. Just take care not to sunburn the scalp.

HAIR COLOR

Let's say dandruff isn't your problem. Maybe you just hate the color of your hair. One of the main reasons for coloring hair is **graying**. When hair turns gray it can also take on a yellowish tone. If you're starting to gray, check your diet. **Inositol** is vital for hair growth. Drinking heavy amounts of caffeine may cause a shortage of inositol in the body. Eat more fruits, vegetables, whole grains, meat and dairy products.
    Supplementing the diet with **PABA** may also restore gray hair to its natural color, if graying was caused by stress or a nutritional

deficiency. PABA can be found in liver, molasses and whole grain foods.

Maybe you've tried the diet route and you're still gray. No sweat. Just give some of these recipes a try:

Elderberry Dye

Elderberries
Water
Heat elderberries in water until just boiling. Allow to steep until cool. Strain out berries. Use the juice to color hair. Dilute juice if necessary to avoid purple hair. Works best for dark hair.

Sage Hair Dye

Sage leaves
Water
Follow the directions for Elderberry Dye. Also works best for dark hair.

Green Oil Dye

Elderberry leaves
Linseed oil
Flax oil
Boil one part leaves to 3 parts linseed and flax oil. Allow to cool and strain. Has been used for centuries to dye hair.

Brunette and Redhead Rinse

Walnut shells
Henna
Water
Cook walnut shells in water and mix a little red henna into it for a lovely, soft red-brown color. This works better for graying redheads than straight henna, which will turn hair carrot-red.

HAIR LOSS

Perhaps the only thing worse than a bad hair day is the fear of a no-hair day. The sales of Rogaine (minoxidil) have skyrocketed since the product was introduced to the market. Minoxidil started out as a blood-pressure medication, but patients often found themselves growing hair while undergoing treatment. While it has been shown to work in some cases, most people see no improvement. Rogaine has to be taken faithfully, forever. For those who achieve some re-growth, it takes up to six months to get any results and the hair is usually extremely fine and sparse.

Not covered by most insurance plans, Rogaine can be an expensive option. My husband tried it in '90 and it was $60 for a two-month supply. After nearly a year of treatment, the results were negligible. Now, if I were balding, no amount of money would seem unreasonable to keep my hair. Unfortunately, there is nothing on the market that really works at any price.

There are, however, herbal remedies which CAN make a difference and cost little more than your time.

Cayenne pepper is used as a hair-restorer. Apply the pepper to your scalp as often as possible. Beware of getting cayenne in your eyes! It won't cause any real damage, but believe me, it will feel like it does! Just don't forget it's up there.

Another way to apply cayenne is as follows:

Vodka Hair Thickener

4 oz. 100 proof vodka
1 tbls. cayenne pepper

Mix vodka and pepper. Refrigerate overnight and strain through cheesecloth. Use a Q-tip to massage the amber-colored liquid on the scalp where hair is thin. Growth will be stimulated.

Keep an eye to your diet and stress level. My husband found that working long hours and stress accelerated his hair loss.

To those with long hair: it's not a myth that ponytails cause baldness. Tight braids and ponytail styles can cut off circulation and bring on a receding hairline. Never wear tight hairstyles and alternate styles, allowing hair to move freely.

Remember, the best hair style is one your hair follows naturally. Work with your hair's natural tendencies and in the long run, your hair will benefit.

> *"Even our enemy is entirely motivated by the quest for happiness. We must recognize that all human beings want the same thing we want."*—Dalai Lama XIV

$\mathcal{H}$OW TO $\mathcal{G}$ET THE $\mathcal{L}$EAD $\mathcal{O}$UT

By Dick Quinn

*L*ead poisoning is a particularly troubling problem because it so often happens to the young and the disadvantaged. It causes dreadful brain damage, learning disabilities and behavior problems. There is an answer, however. There are herbs and other natural substances that remove lead and other heavy metals from the body.

Buckthorn Bark *(Rhamnus frangula)*—taken as a tea, it cleanses lead from the intestine. It is a mild purgative, not to be confused with the laxative Cascara Segrada, which is also called Buckthorn. The tea is available in health stores under the Seelect brand. Herbalists suggest one or two cups per day (morning and afternoon, or evening) for 7 to 10 days.

Onion and **Garlic**—both of these herbs remove lead from the system, whether taken singly or together. Kyolic, a deodorized aged garlic product, has been shown effective in studies.

European studies also prove garlic's cleansing power. Onions, which are closely related to garlic, have been used by herbalists to combat lead poisoning for years. Both are wonderful for the cardiovascular system.

Distilled Water—since it is mineral-free, it leaches iron, lead and other metals from the body. **Note:** people with glaucoma should not drink distilled water.

Apple Pectin—Wash apples, but do not peel because the pectin is just under the skin. Apple pectin helps the body eliminate lead, mercury and other heavy metals. It can be bought in health food stores. Sunflower seeds are another rich source of natural pectin. Synthetic pectin will not work.

Kelp—Kelp is a sea vegetable that protects against radiation, as it removes heavy metals from the body. High in iodine; good for the cardiovascular system.

These herbs are all available in capsules and/or teas from health stores at this time. For dosage, follow the directions on the label and increase the dose in cases of severe poisoning. They are all non-toxic, overdose safe and easy to take singly or together.

How to Rid Your Home of Pests—Safely

By Kelly Quinn

For some parts of the country, autumn means cool temperatures and the end of annoying insects until spring. For others, particularly in the South and West, the bug problem reaches its peak.

The problem arises when life outdoors becomes less attractive to insects than life indoors. As temperatures change, pests look for shelter. It's no surprise they follow you inside.

Insects aren't the only refugees attempting to take up residence in your home. Rodents are also looking for a hospitable place to spend the winter.

How do you eradicate these life-forms without eradicating your own? Pesticides and poisons work great, but the big drawback is that they are poison. Poisons usually work equally well on any life form.

Consider: of 47 different pesticides used by the Los Angeles Unified School District in the '90-'91 school year, 11 were known carcinogens, 27 can cause nerve or genetic damage and three can cause birth defects.

Most pesticides stay active long after the odor dissipates. This residual action is the reason they're so effective. Anything that claims to "keep on killing" for any length of time can be especially dangerous to your health, as well as to the bugs'.

So what's a person to do? A live and let live attitude is not possible in most cases. Insects and rodents spread disease and can cause severe damage to homes. Roach droppings are a leading source of allergy-related asthma. The hantavirus in the Southwest is thought to be spread by rodent droppings.

Fortunately, there are natural, safe methods of pest control. Before you dash out for a can of Raid, try some of these:

The first line of defense is a strong offense. **Caulk holes and cracks** where pests enter. A mouse can get through a hole the size of a pencil. Rats are determined climbers. Look over the outside of your home, from top to bottom, and seal any entry-points. Steel wool is great for blocking holes too big to caulk and rodents can't chew through it.

Keep pet food in a sealed container. Don't let it sit around uneaten as it draws insects and rodents like a magnet. Put giant-size bags in a plastic trash can, covering it with a lid.

Keep dry food in sealed containers. Use old coffee cans with lids, plastic oatmeal containers, or anything that can't be chewed through. Store rice, cereal, dry mixes, sugar, flour and candy this way. Flour and sugar can also be kept in the refrigerator or freezer, if you have extra room. Keep crumbs wiped up, so they won't attract pests.

Sprinkle talcum powder, boric acid, or diatomaceous earth as a border to stop insects. Effective on roaches, ants and termites, diatomaceous earth works like microscopic pieces of sharp glass on insect's bodies. It cuts them and they die. They also take it back to the nest, killing off their friends. It is completely safe for both humans and animals. I use it around my dog's water dish and dog food dish. I put it on my dog, to stop fleas.

Brewer's yeast pills mixed with pet food will discourage bugs from burrowing in its fur. Beware of using flea collars and sprays on your pet. Most don't work and have been known to kill smaller animals. I've seen fleas crawling on flea collars.

However, a **flea collar in your vacuum cleaner bag** is a good idea. When you vacuum, you may vacuum up flea eggs which hatch and are then released into your rug the next time you vacuum. The flea collar will kill any little fleas. It's also a good idea to change the bag frequently.

Wash your pets bedding frequently as well. Simply running the bedding through the dryer on the hot setting will remove and kill fleas and eggs.

Alcohol kills bugs on plants, but it can be tough on the plant. Try **household detergent**, sprayed lightly on plants to discourage bug infiltration.

Bay leaves deter insects. Just spread some around the bug's favorite areas. Make sure kids can't get to it though. **Cucumber rinds** drive away ants and other insects. So does any kind of **mint**.

Common household products often deter ants. **Scrubbing Bubbles**, the foam bathroom cleaner and **hair spray** have been known to turn the tide on an ant invasion and are infinitely less toxic than ant poisons. If you discover an ant attack, try something new. At the very least, you'll wind up with a spotless bathroom. It's also an interesting way to see what the common products we use can do to the environment.

What do you do, despite your best efforts, if you discover a rodent has taken up residence in your house? Traps are your best bet. Poison works, but it can poison other animals and people. Plus it has to be the most interesting thing the rodent can eat, which is rarely the case.

When I was a kid, my dad used to mix up a **Draino sandwich**, which you can try if you are *absolutely sure no living creature can get at it*. It's just what the name describes, Draino on bread, mixed with a little peanut butter. This is extremely toxic. It can also lead to a rather disgusting result. The rodent tends to die quickly, often behind walls, under bathtubs and other places where you can't remove the corpse. After a few days, anyone who enters your house will know it's there, believe me!

Much better than the old Draino sandwich are a bunch of traps. They're cheap and very effective. Use **peanut butter**, old **Easter candy** (the chewy, sugary kind) or **raisins** to bait the traps. Put them where they are easily accessible to rodents and watch the fun. Usually around midnight you'll hear the snapping begin.

Never use the same trap over again. Even if you're brave and can remove the carcass, don't do it. Traps are cheap and rodents spread disease, even dead ones. Just scoop it into a plastic bag and dispose of it in the trash. I use a stick to push it in the bag, so my hands need never touch the trap.

While you're down at the hardware store, they may try to sell you the new thing in rodent control: glue traps. Don't waste your money. I tried them because I thought I could avoid the risk of a trap snapping shut on my fingers. Not only are they expensive, they don't work.

In California, we have a problem with roof rats. They love to climb and a couple had decided the patio roof outside my bedroom window would be the perfect place to make a home. Since my screen had been removed and I couldn't get it back on, I was concerned they'd decide my bedroom was an even better place to live. I put out the traps and went to bed.

Around 1:00 a.m. I was awakened by something banging on the roof outside my window. As I crept to the window to look, a hideous squealing, not unlike that of a pig, arose. Then there was all sorts of banging and crashing around, and I admit, I was afraid to look. I fled downstairs for the rest of the night.

The next morning, I found the traps were torn to shreds, with bunches of hair stuck to them. Apparently, all they did was infuriate the rats. All the bait had been eaten too. That day, I bought some traps. No one has designed a better mousetrap!

It was actually a relief the glue traps didn't work. All they'd do is stop the rat, they wouldn't kill it. What in the world would I have done with an enraged rat? No, traps are definitely the way to go.

I hope these tips will help you win the war on pests. As far as the two-legged kind, you're on your own.

---

*K*EEP *Y*OUR *P*ROSTATE *H*EALTHY... *N*ATURALLY

By Dick Quinn

*P*rostate problems from simple irritation to full blown cancer afflict a growing number of American men. Surgery and other drastic measures risk impotence, incontinence—even death. As Hypocrites said, "Above all, do no harm," so let's try the safest methods first—especially since they work.

Pumpkin seeds (*preferably raw*) are prescribed for a healthy prostate by virtually every herbalist. They're especially high in zinc and are sold in any quantity. You can eat them as a snack.

Parsley eases urination and is an ideal diuretic. You can eat some with every meal, drink it as a tea or take it in capsules.

Small flowered willow herb is the big hit for prostate treatment in Europe. Drink it as a tea—three cups per day until the condition is corrected, then tow cups per day as a maintenance tea. Look for it in health stores. To learn more about it, see Maria Treben's book *Health Through God's Pharmacy*, page 39. She also recommends it for bladder and kidney problems and for prostate cancer.

Stinging nettle juice—research conducted in Germany has shown the juice effective in treating enlarged prostate.

Saw palmetto berry reduces inflammation, pain and throbbing. It is recommended for all glandular problems. It can be taken as a tea or in capsules. Get it in health stores or from the palm.

Cornsilk is a diuretic like parsley and is recommended for bladder infections, as well as prostate. Get it at the health store, grocery store or corn field.

Buchu leaf is a urinary disinfectant that can be taken as tea or in capsules. Originally discovered by the Hotentots of South Africa, who call it Bookoo, it is used for diseases of the kidney, bladder and prostate.

Kelp is used throughout Asia to treat kidney, bladder, prostate and uterine problems. Clinical research shows that, taken daily, kelp reduces prostate swelling in older men to a point where urination becomes painless. It's also a blood cleaner with antibiotic properties. Get it at the health store or sea shore.

July 1993

Dear Reader,

When something saves your life, it gets your attention. That's why I feel so strongly about Cayenne Red Pepper. That wonderful stuff has kept me alive for nearly 15 years.

Cayenne does so much, it's almost unbelievable. In fact, it was unbelievable to a friend of mine. I remember his laughing skepticism when I told him about it in 1987. He was HIV positive and I thought it might help forestall the onset of AIDS. We never found out. He died a few weeks ago.

Herbalists use Cayenne to treat acne and other skin problems, improve appetite, treat arteriosclerosis, arthritis, asthma, bronchitis, colds, colitis, convulsions, cough, cramps, diabetes, and digestive disorders.

I have found Cayenne regulates my blood pressure. It cleans my arteries and other circulatory channels by removing dead fibrin and other deposits that impede blood flow. Dr. John Christopher used Cayenne to treat childhood diseases, flu, gas and hay fever. It stops bleeding instantly. Just try it on a shaving cut. Cayenne kills pain and bacteria to promote faster healing.

Since Cayenne destroys the dead blood cells that cause harmful blood clots, it prevents strokes and heart attacks, while it opens arteries to aid kidney function and help the lung oxygenate the blood. Herbalists also use it to prevent and treat migraine headaches. It helps the pancreas and spleen.

A friend found Cayenne gave him relief from Crohn's disease, when nothing else would. It clears sinus congestion, alleviates shock, heals ulcers, treats yeast infections, hemorrhoids and varicose veins. It even warms cold hands and feet. I have put it in my shoes to keep my feet warm in the Minnesota winter.

It's a circulatory herb, it's a respiratory herb, it's a digestive herb. Cayenne is just too good to be true, but it is true. It really works. Just put it in your body and you'll see. My daily dose is 6 capsules, but most people only need 3 or 4.

I haven't had the flu since I started taking Cayenne in 1978; I never have a headache or constipation. It's wonderful to wake up every day full of energy and feeling terrific.

Cayenne has made life worth living. I have completely escaped the nightmare blood pressure drugs, heart suppressors and blood thinners that make so many good people depressed, impotent, chemical dependents. Cayenne prevents fatigue and depression for me, I bet it will for you, too. Best of all, it works as well today as it did when I first took it October 20, 1978, after my heart attack.

Cayenne is my miracle and I'm telling everyone. I hope you will tell everyone, too. It's vital we spread the word about this wonderful herb, while it's legal without prescription.

We have to help each other help ourselves to health.

Take care of yourself,

Dick Q.

P.S. I was told Cayenne is No. 2 on the FDA hit list—B_6 is No. 1.

$\mathcal{H}$ow to $\mathcal{H}$elp $\mathcal{Y}$ourself $\mathcal{H}$eal $\mathcal{S}$ports $\mathcal{I}$njuries

By Kelly Quinn

*M*y eleven-year-old son hurt his foot right at the beginning of summer. I don't know if he fell off his bike or what, but for weeks he was gimping around and could barely move his ankle.

After a few weeks it seemed he was on the mend, then he stepped in a hole and the problem became chronic. Nothing was broken, he just complained that it hurt if he put pressure on it. We thought maybe he'd sprained it.

Months passed and the poor kid was still walking like he had a wooden leg. He was upset, talking wistfully of being like other boys, able to run and ride his bike without pain.

I gave him some tea to detox him. He drank it, but it didn't help. One day his grandpa saw him gimping around and said it looked like he had gout. Grandpa would know, because he suffers from gout occasionally.

So Grandpa (Dick Quinn, in case you hadn't guessed) made Quinn (my son) some Gout Caps. Quinn tried them and was amazed, they worked! And they worked fast, by the second day Quinn said there was no pain. He was thrilled!

While visiting some relatives, Quinn ran out of his Gout Caps. His ankle started hurting again. At dinner with the family one night, he announced that he had gout. Everyone exploded into laughter to hear an eleven year old say he had gout, a condition usually associated with Henry the VIII.

But, we got the kid more caps and sure enough, they worked. I don't know if he really had gout, but to him, it doesn't matter. He found something that made him feel like himself again.

I think he had an injury to his ankle that became a chronic condition. A lot of people have old injuries that become chronic. A sprain that never quite goes away, a bum knee, tennis elbow, a sore wrist. I suspect if I'd taken him in for a thorough examination (I did have the doctor look at it while he was getting stitches out) they'd have said he had some sort of arthritic condition, given him some aspirin and sent him on his way. But, that wouldn't have taken care of the problem.

The kid is eleven. I don't want him to be doomed to anti-inflammatories for the rest of his life. None of them are without side-effects, especially taken over a long period of time.

And it's not uncommon for an injury to become arthritic or to develop bursitis. It happens to lots of people. If it happens to you or someone you know, why not give Quinn's Gout Caps a try? You can't buy them, but you can make them. Here's the recipe:

Quinn's Gout Caps

2 parts Safflower
2 parts Queen of the Meadow, also known as Gravelroot
1 part Celery Seed
1 part Burdock
1 part Chickweed

A "part" can be any measurement, as long as they are equal. You can use a teaspoon, a tablespoon, ¼ cup measure (you'll make a lot), it doesn't matter. Throw the parts in a blender and grind it up until the consistency is uniform. Don't put it on liquefy! Fill gelatin capsules with the mix. You can get them at the drugstore. If you don't want to use capsules, you can flatten some bread and make a little burrito. You can also put it on your salad, if you want (although burdock is pretty bitter).

Take about 3 caps twice a day to start. Then about three a day until you are healed. Use how you feel as a gauge. Quinn starts with more, then tapers off.

It's also a good idea to work the injured area if you can. This recipe should be good for arthritis as well, as burdock and celery seed are herbs for the treatment of arthritis. Cherries are another thing to try. You can eat maraschino cherries, cherry pie, cherry juice or raw cherries, just bulk up on the cherries.

Don't let the name of the caps put you off. What you have may not really be gout (high levels of uric acid, usually due to improper eating habits, but possibly injury). If you're a kid, you don't care what it is, you just want it gone.

Out of the mouths of babes...

How to Face the Flu Season

By Kelly Quinn

The beginning of the new school year coincides with the onset of the cold and flu season. Here are some tips and natural remedies that should make illnesses more tolerable and less frequent.

Don't hesitate to increase your vitamin C intake at the first sign of illness. Be sure children get extra C as well, but keep it to 500 mg. as a supplement for kids. More may result in diarrhea, which is a problem your kids don't need. At the first sign of a cold I give my kids an extra C in the morning and often at dinner as well. When you feel confident they are healthy, cut back. I found that upping the vitamin C in such a fashion helped my kids avoid many of the debilitating colds and flu viruses that struck down most of the kids in our neighborhood.

Give zinc a try. It tastes horrible, even the flavored versions taste like metallic chalk, but it does seem to work. At the first sign of illness, or when you are ill and can bear it no longer, suck a zinc. It doesn't help to swallow a supplement as the body does not absorb it a well as when it is allowed to dissolve in the mouth. Get the cheap, low dosage kind, forget about time-release types and capsules. As the zinc dissolves, swish it around in your mouth so it coats everything but your teeth. It's repulsive, but hey, it works.

Wash your hands. Most viruses are passed by touching something a virus-ridden person has come in contact with. Door knobs, light switches, telephones, magazines, etc. can all be contaminated. Viruses don't live long on objects, but it doesn't take much time to pass illnesses along in a busy household or office. Ideally, people who are ill should wash their hands every time they touch their eyes, mouth, or blow their nose. Let's face it, that just doesn't happen. So, when someone is sick, everyone should become obsessed with hand washing for a while.

Try a dragon cocktail. At the first sign of a stuffy nose, dry, or itchy throat, or anything that doesn't feel right, mix about a teaspoonful of cayenne pepper in a glass of tomato juice and drink up. The more it sits, the hotter it gets, so don't try to make up a vat the night before. Add garlic and onion to boost the medicinal effects as nature's antibiotic. During a cold, regular dragon cocktails will keep the sinuses much clearer than conventional cold medicines (which have been shown to be ineffective in children under 12), will eliminate a hacking cough, and act as a natural expectorant. It will also give you the thrill of feeling normal for a few hours. Kids like them too. I can't keep tomato juice in the house, as the kids are always making up dragon cocktails.

Take a steam bath. Turn the shower on hot, lock the bathroom door and settle in to suck up some steam. It loosens congestion in the chest and sinuses and gets the crud moving again, lessening the chances of a simple cold turning into bronchitis or a sinus infection. Sit there as long as possible, 20 minutes is ideal. Don't sit in the shower as it will be too hot. Just have a seat on the commode and catch up on your reading.

Invest in a vaporizer. The debate has raged for years over which is best: hot vaporizers or cold ones. The cold ones win. Hot vaporizers are an ideal environment for bacteria. Cool vapor can help shrink swollen, congested tissues and ease breathing. The idea is to keep the air moist while the ill person recuperates.

Drink, drink, and drink some more. Lots of juice, water, and tea. Stay away from milk, as it can add to mucus. Tea made with licorice root contains a natural chemical that enables throat membranes to secrete moisture and eliminate mucus. Teas containing chickweed, fenugreek, comfrey root, and slippery elm are also excellent for colds.

Suck on some candy. Sugars are demulcents, a substance that coats the back of the throat and subdues the sensation that leads to coughing. Hard candies made from real licorice root (not anise, which is used in most licorice made in this country, you'll have to shop around) help to ease a sore throat. Eucalyptus or mentholated candies can really help ease congestion and breathing.

Gargle with salt water. Use hot water, 1/2 teaspoon salt to 8 ounces water, four times a day. This washes away mucus and dilates capillaries in the throat, increasing the blood supply to the area which brings more antibodies to fight the infection. Do not over or under salt the water, as too little or too much could increase irritation.

Eat lots of chicken soup. Studies have shown that chicken soup works better than mere warm water at clearing out congestion and easing symptoms. Put some garlic, red pepper and onions in it and you'll have the perfect infection fighting meal.

Make lemonade. Lemons are natural decongestants and supply lots of vitamin C. To rid your body of the by-products of illness, you need lots of fluid. Lemonade flavored with sugar or honey soothes a sore throat.

Upset stomach? Sip a room temperature glass of ginger ale or lemon lime soda. If you can, let it go flat first. This helps neutralize stomach acids and prevent you from becoming dehydrated. The sugar (pass on diet drinks for the time being) gives your body a bit of energy, which it needs to get well. Ginger calms an upset stomach.

Feeling a trifle gaseous? Brew up a batch of peppermint tea. Peppermint contains natural chemicals that break up and expel intestinal gas. Chamomile tea is good for stomach aches, especially in children.

How do you stop diarrhea? When someone is troubled by diarrhea, he should stick to a low fiber diet for a couple days and heavy up on white rice and bananas. The starch in the rice acts as a thickening agent, if you know what I mean. Bananas are high in potassium. The old standby, Kaopectate works pretty well and there are many new remedies on the market, all of which are very high-priced. Red raspberry leaf is a heck of a lot cheaper and works just as well. It is also high in vitamin C and can be used to alleviate the problems of PMS and other women's difficulties. You can't say that for good old Kaopectate. Raspberry leaves are difficult to encapsulate, but work well as tea or eaten mixed in foods. They don't have much taste and certainly not an unpleasant one. Other herbs for diarrhea include barberry, garlic, goldenseal, and slippery elm. Make sure the patient gets plenty of fluids, as diarrhea is very dehydrating.

Get some fresh air. The stale, canned air in most houses and offices in the winter encourages illness. There have been reports of people who keep their bedroom windows open year round and never get colds. Taken with a grain of salt (as most reports should be), it makes sense to breathe fresh air whenever possible. Ever notice how you feel better when you go outside when you have a cold? Give it a shot.

Get into the zen of illness. The watery eyes, stuffy nose and crud in your chest are the way your body is trying to eliminate the bugs. Your body knows what it's doing. Don't get in its way, help it work by drinking and eating good things and getting lots of rest.

If, despite your best intentions, you still find yourself sick, relax. Following these hints should at least lessen the duration and minimize the pain of the illness. It's important to regain your strength so you can fight off the next bug that comes around.

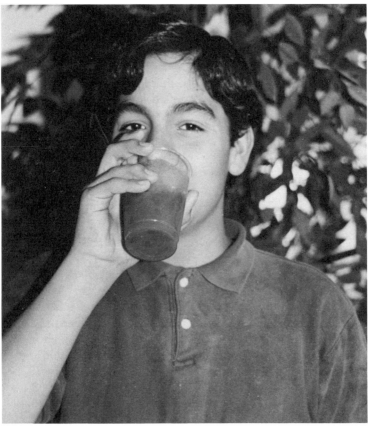

One cayenne dragon cocktail and Matt's sore throat goes up in flames.

*H*ELP *Y*OURSELF *S*OOTHE AN *U*PSET *S*TOMACH

By Kelly Quinn

I never used to be troubled with stomach problems, in fact, I thought I had a cast-iron stomach. I could eat anything and everything (and frequently did). I never bought Rolaids or Tums. If I bought Pepto-Bismal, it was in case one of the kids needed it, and I usually threw it away unused after the expiration date on the bottle.

I didn't even know what half the products on the market for stomach problems were for. Then, I found out I had hepatitis last year and embarked upon an unpleasant journey of discovery through the drugstore.

I was troubled by flatulence (a word that used to make me chuckle, until it became a problem for me and I found it no laughing matter), nausea, acidity, sour stomach you name it. There are so many products out there at a wide range of prices and what works one day, may not work the next.

An occasional side-effect of some remedies is constipation. I sure didn't want to have to deal with that, either. I didn't want to have to deal with any of it, to tell you the truth. I started treating my formerly cast-iron stomach with kid gloves, ever on the alert for signs of something amiss.

I started carrying an arsenal of remedies with me. I always had an antacid/anti-gas remedy in my purse. I took Tagamet, I started to swig repulsive tasting concoctions.

Then, I went to a health food convention. I saw people shilling aloe juice. Of course, they couldn't tell me what it was for, but it was an interesting concept.

I was on my way home, about two hours away, when my stomach started to bother me. I felt around in my purse for some Mylanta. I was out. As each mile passed, the pain increased. It felt like my stomach was scraped and raw, internally. By the time I got home, I had to go lie down.

The next day I had a million things to do and my stomach started acting up as soon as I got on the road. It still felt sore, and I tried to think of what I could take that would be soothing. Then I remembered the aloe juice. I'd gotten a few samples and given most of them to the kids when they had tummy-aches and it seemed to work. The time seemed ripe for an experiment of my own.

I found a sample bottle and took a swig. It was cranberry flavored, not bad. Within a few minutes, I realized my stomach felt better. A half hour later, I had forgotten all about my troubles. The next day, I went out and bought a jug of the stuff.

It cost about $10 for a quart. I made sure to get one that said it contained active enzymes. I also made sure to get one that was flavored. The clerk at the health-food store said it didn't taste bad plain, but I figured if it was so palatable there wouldn't be the proliferation of flavored varieties. She also said it is used for arthritis, but since I don't have that yet, I can't experiment with its effectiveness there.

Now, I take nothing else for any type of stomach upset. It seems to work quickly and rarely do I need a second dose. What I particularly like is that I don't have to worry about overdosing, or putting a certain time limit between doses. If I get a twinge of stomach pain or upset, I take a swig. If I get another a while later, I take another.

The week after I bought my jug, my kids started coming down with a stomach flu. I gave them only aloe when they complained and it seemed to alleviate nausea, gas and diarrhea. I've heard of those who use it for constipation as well. Barb (a frequent contributor to In Depth) tried it herself and on her kids with the same positive results.

There are, of course, many natural remedies to stomach ailments. If you're not inclined to invest in a jug of aloe juice, or can't get to a health-food store, you may want to try some of these:

Red Raspberry Tea. Pour one cup boiling water over four to five leaves. Cover and steep for 10 minutes. Strain and sweeten to taste.

Ginger. Take two or three gelatin capsules of powdered ginger root.

Accupressure. Firmly press the area between your thumb and index finger. Press hard and rub in a circular motion for several minutes. This works well in cases of mild nausea and even for headaches.

Horseradish. If you suffer from indigestion and eat a lot of beef, add horseradish to your diet. Horseradish helps you digest red meat. Rosemary aids in the digestion of lamb and fennel may work for oily fish.

For a digestive tonic: Stir one tablespoon ground aniseed into one cup of milk. Drink twice daily.

Oatmeal. Chew a teaspoon of dry rolled oats and then swallow them.

Peppermint Tea is highly recommended for any digestive disorder. Cold sage tea, made by pouring one quart of boiling water over two ounces honey and one ounce bruised sage leaves is also used to relieve gas. Cover and steep the tea for several hours, then refrigerate.

Caraway, fennel and thyme teas are also recommended for stomach ailments.

Slippery Elm is an herb you should always have on the shelf. It is used for a variety of ailments, from wounds, sore throats and coughs, to bronchial congestion. It's used as a laxative and to treat diarrhea. It's good for ulcers, and soothing to a sore stomach. To make tea, boil from one to three tablespoonful of powdered bark in one cup of water. Let it simmer 15 minutes. Drink up to three cups per day. You can sweeten if you like. Very palatable herb, you can even get kids to take it. You can also take it in capsule form.

Catnip is not only for cats. It works for nausea, cramps, spasms, gas and nervous disorders. It helps in digestion as well.

Chamomile tea was what Peter Rabbit had when he ate too many cabbages. You might want to give that a try as well. If you are treating a child, it's a good idea to read them the story of Peter Rabbit while they sip their tea. Chamomile also acts as a natural sedative to induce sleep, so don't be surprised if your young patient falls asleep before Peter makes it home.

To aid digestion and perhaps prevent future problems, eat more **Papaya** and **Pineapple**. Chronic indigestion calls for major lifestyle changes. Start exercising, if you don't already. Drink at least eight glasses of water per day. Water helps you digest the bulky fibers that are so important to the health of the intestinal tract. Be sure to include a selection of whole grains, fruits, and vegetables in your daily diet to keep fiber at an adequate level.

Smoking can aggravate heartburn and indigestion. Alcohol can inflame the stomach lining. Learn to relax. Sleep on an extra pillow to raise your upper body a bit, this can alleviate nocturnal heartburn.

Most of the over-the-counter remedies are mild and work well. They can be prohibitively expensive and should not be taken regularly. Pepto-Bismal type medications should not be taken with any aspirin based medications, as it can combine with the salicylic acid and cause a ringing in the ears. Since these aren't things you have to worry about with the natural remedies listed, it makes sense to look into them before purchasing an over-the-counter medication.

Help Yourself Stop Yeast Infections

By Kelly Quinn

Women are forced to undergo many unpleasantries due solely to gender. Vaginal yeast infections are among the most distressing and irritating "femal problems."

Yeast infections are increasingly common complaints as evidenced by the proliferation of advertising for over-the-counter remedies. In the days before man-made fabrics, showers and antibiotics, yeast infections were much less common. Tight clothing, underwear of man-made fibers, quick showers, stress and the use of antibiotics can also trigger a yeast infection.

Antiobiotics kill the "friendly" bacteria that keep yeast growth under control. Nylon underwear doesn't allow the area to "breathe," encouraging the growth of "unfriendly" bacteria. Douching is an unnecessary practice and can wash out needed friendly bacteria. Showers do fine at cleaning the exterior but little towards cleansing the genital area properly.

Itching, burning upon urination and increased discharge are symptomatic of yeast infections. For a precise diagnosis, a visit to the doctor's office is a good idea as there are many different vaginal infections, some of which can result in sterility if left untreated.

If you're familiar with the symptoms of a yeast infection, you can try the over-the-counter medication which usually works. It can be rather expensive, however, costing upwards of $12 for a week's supply. Most of the brands are equally effective, containing the same active ingredient.

There are alternatives to pharmaceuticals, some of which you may already have around the house.

For quick relief of symptoms, try a **sitz bath**. Fill a tub with warm water, deep enough to cover the affected area. Add either ½ cup salt or ½ cup vinegar. Sit in the water for at least 10 minutes.

Also worth a try is applying **plain yogurt** with active cultures directly to the affected area. To put "good" bacteria back into your system, drink **acidophilis milk or** eat **yogurt** with acidophilis cultures. If you suffer from recurrent yeasts infections, this should lessen their frequency.

If you're into **tea**, you can try an herb tea made from **blue flag, echinachea, periwinkle, St. Johns' wort** and **white deadnettle**. You should drink the tea three times a day for up to six weeks as a time.

An unusual but extremely effective remedy is to insert a whole clove of **garlic**, peeled without scraping the surface and dipped in olive oil, into the vagina overnight. This can help clear up symptoms if tried early.

Tree tea oil is an effective anti-fungal that does not irritate the vaginal membranes. Dilute 5 ml. oil in 15 ml. carrier oil and put 5 drops on a tampon. Insert for 4 hours. You can also try it in suppositories or cream.

Pot marigold or **calendula** officianalis is anti fungal, astringent, and very healing. You can put some in the bath and soak in it or try douching with a tea.

Other herbs to try are: **buchu, white oak bark** and **pau d'arco.**

To discourage future yeast infections, wear looser clothing, use only cotton underwear, avoid douching and feminine deodorant products (unnecessary if personal hygiene is not neglected; in fact if a deodorant is needed, that is a sign of infection). Stay away from deodorant tampons and pads (the yeast infection symptoms could be a sign of sensitivity to the fragrance). Don't use powder (starch promotes bacteria growth). Always urinate before and after intercourse to flush germs out of the uretha.

Some people are sensitive to yeasts and processed sugars in foods. If you get frequent yeast infections, try a yeast and sugar-free diet for a cople of weeks and monitor your progress. You may find yourself free of symptoms until you increase yoru intake of yeasts. Undertaking a yeast-free diet is an education in itself. You'll be amazed at how many foods contain yeast and yeast extract. You'll probably lose a bit of weight if you stay yeast-free for a while.

If, despite your best efforts to avoid one, you find yourself with a yeast infection, try this to prevent re-infection: touch the crotch of your underwear with a hot iron to kill any residual bacteria that may not have been removed in the wash. Do this on clean underwear only! Also, do not try this on underwear made of anything other than cotton, as nylon and polyester melt when heat is applied.

If your infection does not go away, or appears to worsen, you may have more than a simple yeast infection. In which case, a visit to the doctor is required for proper diagnosis and treatment options.

HELP YOURSELF LEARN TO USE HERBS

By Kelly Quinn

Herbs are wonderful foods to use for good health and healing. But, it can be confusing when trying to figure out exactly how best to use them. What is an infusion, decoction, or tincture, anyway? How do you make one? We're going to clear up some of those questions and answer a few others, like: what's the difference between an extract or whole herb? Which is better?

The first thing you should do is go out and pick up a good book on herbs. There are many. If you've been a regular reader of *Help Yourself To Health,* you know we often recommend books. No matter how much you know about herbs, questions always arise.

There are bizillions of herb books out there. What you want is a relatively cheap one that contains many herbs and their uses. You can find one that even details how to make various herbal mixtures. Some of my personal favorites are: *The Complete Medicinal Herbal* by Penelope Ody. It retails for $29.95, which is a bit too rich for my blood, but I picked it up for $13.95 at a discount store. It has many color pictures and is a wonderful resource. I also like *Prescription For Nutritional Healing* by James F. Balch, M.D. and Phyllis A. Balch, C.N.C. It retails for $16.95. Louis Tenney's *Health Handbook* is an excellent book to take with you everywhere. It retails for $5.95 and is smaller than a paperback, but packs a wealth of information and recipes into 331 pages.

Don't overlook the el cheapo books at the grocery store check stands. For 89¢ each, I got *The Magic of Nature's Healing Herbs* and *Natural Health Remedies*. I use these two little books all the time. They touch on a myriad of ailments and provide common sense, easy-to-find remedies.

Check out discount bookstores for herb books. Also used bookstores and libraries have some bargains. What's great about old herb books is they never go out of date. Herbs and their applications have been around for centuries. The older books are often more valuable than the new ones.

So, let's say you have a problem. You looked up the herbs to try and you're on the way to the health store to pick them up. As you stand among the dizzying array of choices, the question looms: which is better, whole herb or extract?

Check your resource first to see if it mentions which part of the herb to use. A basic rule of thumb is that whole herbs are safer than extracts. Nature provides natural safeguards in herbs to prevent nasty side-effects or overdose. When an extract is made, these natural safeguards may be left out and the active ingredients are concentrated and therefore, stronger. So, whenever possible, get whole herbs, whether powdered, ground, shredded, in leaves or chunks.

Extracts usually come in little bottles of fluid or in pills and are not whole herbs.

Sometimes, though, it is next to impossible to get the herb in any form but an extract, as in the case of lobelia. Get the extract, but use it judiciously. Remember, the strength of the herb has been increased. If your herb book's recipe calls for an extract, don't worry, the strength has already been accounted for.

The next question that usually arises is: How much do I take? Remember, herbs are foods. They are not drugs. You will have a hard time treating yourself if you try to take them as you would a couple of Tylenol. For one thing, they do not come in 250 or 500 mg. sizes. It's also not like taking a 12-hour tiny time pill. Usually, with herbs, you take the tea or capsules a few times a day, because like other food, it passes through your system and out the dumpster. The biggest concern with herbs is not overdosing, but underdosing. Okay, so you've got your herbs and it's time to put something together. First, here's some standard measurements:

You can use standard spoons, droppers or measuring cups for doses. Quantities for infusions and decoctions should be divided into three equal doses.

Drop doses = 5-10 drops depending on age and/or condition.	
1 ml. = 20 drops	65 ml. = ¼ cup
5 ml. = 1 teaspoon	130 ml. = ½ cup
20 ml. = 1 tablespoon	

An **Infusion** is a very simple way of using herbs and is made much the same way as making tea. The water should be just off the boil, since vigorously boiling water disperses valuable volatile oils in the steam. Use this method for flowers and the leafy parts of plants. The standard quantity should be made fresh each day and is sufficient for three doses. Drink hot or cold.

Put the herb in a pot with a close-fitting lid. A teapot is ideal. Pour hot water over the herb. Allow to infuse for 10 minutes, then pour through a nylon sieve or strainer into a teacup. Store the rest in a pitcher in a cool place.

Standard quantities: 30 g. dried herb or 75 g. fresh herb to 500 ml. (about 2 cups) water. Standard dose: one-half cup three times a day.

A **Decoction** involves a more vigorous extraction of a plant's active ingredients than an infusion and is used for roots, barks, twigs and some berries. As with infusions, the standard quantity should be made fresh each day and is enough for three doses. Drink hot or cold.

Place the herb in a saucepan and add cold water. Bring to boil, then simmer for up to one hour until the volume has been reduced by one-third. Strain through a nylon sieve into a pitcher or teacup. Store in a cool place.

Standard quantities: 30 g. dried herb or 60 g. fresh herb to 750 ml. (3 cups) water, reduced to about 500 ml. (2 cups) by simmering. Standard dose: ½ cup, three times a day.

A **Tincture** is made by steeping the dried or fresh herb in a 25% mixture of alcohol and water. Any part of the plant may be used. Besides extracting the plant's active ingredients, the alcohol acts as a preservative and tinctures will keep for up to two years. Tinctures should be made from individual herbs, combine prepared tinctures as required. Commercial tinctures use ethyl alcohol, but diluted spirits are suitable for home use. Vodka is ideal, since it contains few additives, although rum helps to disguise the flavor of less palatable herbs.

Put the herb into a large jar and cover with the vodka/water mixture. Seal the jar, store in a cool place for two weeks and shake it occasionally. Fit cheesecloth around the rim of a wine press, pour the mixture through. Press the mixture through the wine press into a jug. The residue makes excellent compost for your herb garden! Pour the strained liquid into clean, dark glass bottles, using a funnel.

Standard quantities: 200 g. dried herb or 600 g. fresh herb to 1 liter 25% alcohol/water mixture (dilute a 75 cl. bottle of 37.5% vodka with 37.5 ml. water). Standard dose: 5 ml. three times a day. Tinctures should be taken diluted in water (a little honey or fruit juice can often improve the flavor).

REMEMBER! Tinctures contain alcohol which can be detrimental to pregnant women, children, recovering alcoholics, and people with liver disease. To de-alcoholize the tincture, add 25-50 ml. of almost boiling water to the tincture dose in a cup and allow it to cool. This effectively evaporates most of the alcohol.

CAUTION! Do not use industrial alcohol, methylated spirits (methyl alcohol), or rubbing alcohol in tinctures. All are extremely toxic.

A **Syrup** is made with honey or unrefined sugar to preserve infusions and decoctions and makes an ideal cough remedy—honey is particularly soothing. The added sweetness also disguises the flavor of more unpleasant-tasting herbs, such as motherwort. Syrups can also be used to favor medicines for kids.

Heat 500 ml. standard infusion or decoction in a sauce pan. Add 500 g. honey or unrefined sugar and stir constantly until dissolved. allow the mixture to cool and pour into a dark glass bottle. Seal with a cork stopper. Cork is important as syrups often ferment and screw-capped bottles can explode.

Standard quantities: 500 ml. infusion or decoction, 500 g. honey or unrefined sugar. Standard dose: 5-10 ml.; three times a day.

You can extract the active plant ingredients from herbs in oil for external use in massage oils, creams and ointments. Infused oils will last up to a year if kept in a cool, dark place, though smaller amounts made fresh are more potent. There are two techniques, the hot method, suitable for comfrey, chickweed, or rosemary; and the cold method for marigold and St. John's wort. If possible, repeat the process for cold infused oil using new herb and the once-infused oil, leaving to stand for a few more weeks before straining.

Hot Infusion: Put the oil and the herb in a glass bowl over a pan of boiling water or in a double boiler saucepan and heat gently for about three hours. Pour the mixture into a cheesecloth fitted securely to the rim of a wind press and strain into a jug. Pour into clean, airtight storage bottles, using a funnel.

Standard quantities: 250 g. dried herb or 750 g. fresh herb to 500 ml. sunflower oil.

Cold Infusion: Pack a large jar tightly with the herb and cover completely with oil. Put the lid on and leave on a sunny windowsill for two to three weeks. Pour the mixture into a jelly bag or cheesecloth, fitted securely with string or rubber band to the rim of a jug. Squeeze the oil through. Repeat the first two steps with new herb and the once-infused oil, after a few weeks, strain again and store.

Standard quantities: enough flower heads to pack a storage jar, 1 liter cold pressed oil.

Some other ways to take herbs that are very simple are: as steam inhalants, skin washes and drink in juices.

Don't let the metric measurements throw you off, you'll find some of the best herb books come from other countries where the metric system is King. You'll also find that most measuring cups and spoons these days have both the American system of measurement and the metric system. Don't worry about being too precise either. Using herbs is like baking a cake, you need the general idea of how much of what to put in and when. It's not complicated, it's not supposed to be.

Just remember to relax and have a little fun.

August 1993

Dear Reader,

In November 1992, a 44 year-old New York advertising executive in California to visit his retired parents, was awakened from a sound sleep one night when somebody "jumped in my face."

He said the assailant's "hair was long and spikey, and his mouth was melted and burnt and dripping like a mask, like he had a clown suit on."

The man leapt out of bed and attacked the intruder with his fists and a ceramic object, beating him into submission. "I was totally savage, out of my mind," he said. "I went absolutely berserk and just hit him and hit him." Then he called 911, saying he had caught an intruder and reported that his father was missing.

When police arrived, they found his 77 year-old father hog-tied with a phone cord, laying in a pool of blood in the atrium of his home. His skull was split open from his neck to his forehead, his eyes were swollen shut and part of his ear was missing. More than eight months after the attack, he is still in the sub-acute unit of a California hospital, kept alive by machines that feed him and help him breathe. He has been in a coma since the attack.

On August 3rd, after two and a half days of deliberation, a jury of six men and six women acquitted his son of attempted murder and torture by reason of temporary insanity induced by Halcion, an addictive sleep drug manufactured by the Upjohn Company, makers of Zanax. Halcion, which was introduced in 1982, is tied to so many violent acts it is banned in England, France and many other countries, yet it is freely prescribed here.

A Utah woman was acquitted of murder after taking Halcion.

*She shot her mother eight times at midnight on the day before her
83rd birthday, then placed a birthday card in her hands. The jury
found the woman "incapable of voluntary action" because of psychosis induced by Halcion. The FDA approves its continued sale,
making insomnia treatment life threatening to us all.*

*In 1991, the FDA came to my herb company in Minneapolis and
banned sale of a safe, effective herbal sleep formula because it didn't
contain one of two approved chemicals, both of which cause kidney
damage. They were protecting Halcion sales.*

*Ironically, the FDA attacked food supplements and herbs as being
of "questionable safety" and possibly "life threatening." Halcion isn't
merely life threatening, it's proven fatal, yet it is prescribed freely to
millions, so the FDA can better serve its masters at the Upjohn
Company.*

*Your safety, my safety, the poor mother and daughter in Utah
and the father and son in California whose lives are forever ruined
— none of us matter in the FDA's insane frenzy to push drugs. While
claiming to "protect" us, they promote murderous drugs and deprive
us of safe alternatives. Their hypocrisy has no limit.*

*In a report to congress, the FDA complained that many vitamins
and dietary supplements make "unsubstantiated claims" to eradicate tumors, boost immune function and other benefits. Of course
all claims are "unsubstantiated" when you reject mountains of
research and thousands of years of clinical experience. To learn, one
must want to know the truth.*

*They say they don't know if things like cayenne are safe. I know
— why don't they? I also know over 150,000 Americans die every
year from drugs sold by the "ethical" drug companies. Nearly 3,000
Americans die from aspirin alone.*

*The FDA should be searching the world for safe remedies that
help us, rather than pushing murderous money-makers like Halcion
for the drug companies. Maybe someday a miracle will happen, but
in the meantime. . .*

> *Take care of yourself,*
>
> *Dick Q.*

GETTING THROUGH THE CHRISTMAS SEASON

By Kelly Quinn

*T*he Christmas season is fraught with temptations that can blow your diet and exercise plan to smithereens. It is also a time of widespread depression, perhaps due in part to the extra pounds and lack of exercise. It doesn't have to be that way. Read on for ideas that can get you through to the New Year. Maybe this year you won't have to resolve to drop the extra ten pounds

Christmas is a time of partying, eating and drinking too much. It's also the time we tend to stray from our exercise routine. After all, who can find time to exercise when every waking hour is spent scouring stores for those "must have" Christmas gifts, wrapping gifts and recovering from yet another Christmas party hangover?

It gets dark early. It's cold, so you spend time with people who may not make you feel filled with goodwill towards mankind. Now it's time to heavy up on Gota Kola to fight depression, enhance memory, and mental energy. An anti-aging herb, Gotu Kola retards the signs of aging and helps combat stress. Ever notice how old and haggard you look when you're stressed?

Be sure to take your cayenne. It will give you real energy to get through the myriads of tasks each day. It will also help cleanse your system of all the crud you put into it with Christmas cookies, delicious but unhealthful foods, and alcohol. You may want to take a cayenne capsule or drink it in juice two to three times a day. Make sure you take it with food or some sort—not hot soup or coffee! It will also help you get the energy you need to maintain an exercise program.

If you don't exercise, this is the time to start. Get in at least a good 30 minutes of exercise three to four times a week. Exercise plays a huge role in fighting stress. It helps you center yourself and relieves anxiety. While you are exercising, you'll find the solutions to many of the incidentals you've been agonizing about become clearer. Stress lowers your body's immunity; exercise raises it.

Heavy up on the Vitamin C. C helps your body repair itself and strengthens the immune system. It helps you fight off the effects of too little sleep and irregular meals. I heavy up on Vitamin C (at least 5,000 mg daily) whenever I feel stressed. Have you noticed you tend to get the cold or flu that's been going around after a week filled with stress or too much partying? When your body has to fight the effects of what you've been doing to it, it has a harder time keeping illness at bay. You don't have time to be sick with all you have going on!

Start adding garlic and vitamin E to your regimen. Vitamin E works well with C as both are anti-oxidants which rebuild and enhance the immune system. They fight off free radicalsthe crud you ingest which has been linked to cancer. Most of us don't get enough of either vitamin through diet, especially in the winter months when fresh fruit and vegetables are harder to come by. Garlic works to fight illnesses and basically attacks anything harmful to the body. It also helps in regulating blood pressure.

As far as food goes, just think small. Small portions of the special treats of the season won't be as detrimental to your diet as trying to deprive yourself entirely. All too often, we decide we won't eat anything "bad," then we wind up gorging ourselves on all kinds of forbidden foods. Thinking "small" means we can have what we want, just not as much. Therefore, we don't feel deprived or become obsessed with what we can't have.

If you know you are going to be eating some things you usually don't, eat lighter during the day. Don't starve yourself, or you are likely to find your willpower snap somewhere between the cheese slices and the Christmas torte.

Go easy on the alcohol. Try to space your drinks with conversation and food. If you do overindulge, drinking lots of fluids (not coffee) like water or juice will help you avoid a hangover. Much of the unpleasantness of a hangover is brought on by dehydration. Alcohol dehydrates. Coffee makes it worse, as coffee is dehydrating as well. Symptoms of dehydration include: headache, nausea, weakness. Sound like a hangover?

Avoid aspirin, acetaminophen (Tylenol) or ibuprofen when there is alcohol in your system. All react negatively with the alcohol and can cause severe, even fatal-reactions. Instead, try White Willow Bark, nature's aspirin. For upset stomach from overindulgence, drink aloe juice. Eat lightly and drink plenty of fluids. Avoid drinking alcohol when taking any drugs, particularly ulcer drugs (Tagamet, Pepcid, Zantac) or cold drugs. Ulcer drugs can slow the metabolizing of alcohol, meaning the drinks are not processed through your system, so you get drunker. It puts quite a strain on your liver. Cold medicines and alcohol intensify side-effects. You could easily find yourself asleep somewhere instead of enjoying the party. If in doubt, always ask the pharmacist, even if the medicine is over-the-counter. If it isn't safe, don't take it.

Sometimes, with all the whirl of responsibilities and activities, you may find yourself tossing and turning instead of getting the rest you desperately need to face and enjoy the season. Don't drink before bedtime. Alcohol may make you sleepy, but you tend to wake up after a couple of hours, even more tired. Better to take some valerian. It's a natural sedative, stress fighter and even fights irregular heartbeats. Have a couple of capsules about an hour before bedtime. You'll find that not only do you sleep well, you feel rested and won't become addicted. Also try chamomile tea, or teas with sage, catnip or red clover. Celestial Seasonings has a tea called Sleepytime and it really does work. You may want to try Passion Flower as well.

Check your attitude. Are you stressing yourself trying to have a Norman Rockwell Christmas with people you rarely see and don't get along with all that well anyway? Christmas is not the time to try to remake your life. Rather, it's the time to be happy with what you have and try to spread a little joy yourself.

If you feel down because there is no one to share your holiday, be grateful you aren't trapped with a bunch of relatives you never see except on holidays and have nothing in common with anyway. You have the perfect opportunity to give your time to someone less fortunate. If you have time, volunteer to help at a hospice, soup kitchen, send Christmas cards to the lonely or gifts to the needy. Although many people love to volunteer, too few can find time on the big day, since they have families and responsibilities of their own to meet. You are desperately needed.

When I moved to California, my family was all back in Minnesota and Wisconsin. Our first Christmas out here, my daughter asked how it could feel like Christmas without snow, old friends, or family. "Christmas," I said, "is a state of mind." That's true. It's not where you are, but who you are and what you have to give that makes a holiday feel special. If you follow our advice you'll be healthy for the holidays, and have the energy to make this the best holiday season, ever.

Happy Holidays!

October 1993

Dear Reader,

I've been getting a lot of calls and letters from people who are interested in trying herbs. They want to know how much to take, how to take it, and if herbs are safe to take with other drugs.

What's of particular concern to me are those people who put off trying something they are convinced will be good for them unless they can get the strongest stuff. Your body doesn't put itself on hold until your brand comes in. It is busy every single day, dealing with all the things it's got to do.

One example is cayenne. Many people who are prime candidates for heart disease call and ask how to get the hottest cayenne. I ask them what they are taking in the meantime, and they tell me: nothing. They want the hot stuff. They want a big bang.

What they don't realize is that a little of something is infinitely better than nothing at all. I hope they all stay alive long enough to find the products they seek.

Don't take chances. Many people who drop dead of heart attacks planned to stop smoking tomorrow, watch their blood pressure tomorrow, go on that diet tomorrow and get exercising tomorrow. Only problem was, tomorrow didn't come.

Do what you can, today. You body will thank you for it by still being functional, tomorrow.

Take care,

P.S. Remember, herbs tend to work by correcting the condition you needed the drugs for in the first place. You may not need those drugs after awhile when the problem itself has been corrected. Watch yourself. Keep track of your progress and monitor your symptoms. Try to bring your doctor into it if you can.

*H*ELP *Y*OURSELF *H*EAL A *H*EADACHE

By Kelly Quinn

I used to suffer from frequent headaches. Headaches were so common to me, they became a part of life which I stopped questioning. At least once a day, usually in the afternoon, I'd notice a headache and take a pain-reliever. It usually worked. I used pain-relievers with such regularity, I should have been getting thank-you notes from the manufacturers.

Then I developed sinus trouble. I had a headache that simply would not go away. In fact, it got so bad, I was experiencing new levels of pain. Finally, I went to the doctor and he determined I had a sinus infection. After hearing my history, he suggested that I may have allergies, resulting in pressure and congestion which led to my frequent headaches. No, he told me, daily headaches are not normal.

After clearing up the infection and taking decongestants, I found myself headache free. It was delightful to realize I hadn't needed painkillers in days. I found myself wondering: how many people treat the symptoms of a problem, without going after the source, as I did.

Think about it. How many times have you reached for a painkiller or other symptom-relieving medication only to re-experience the same problem mere hours later? Because it is so easy to treat just the symptoms of a problem ourselves, we don't often realize we are doing our health a disservice.

Most headaches are caused by tension, or stress. Many, many are caused by allergies and sinus problems. Some are caused by food allergies. Only rarely does a headache stem from a serious condition, such as a tumor. Some stem from hormonal changes. For example, I will frequently get severe headaches just days before my period.

The first thing to do when you have a headache is take a moment and ask what could be causing it. If you suffer frequent headaches, you should consider keeping a headache diary, detailing what you have eaten, activities you've participated in, weather conditions, and where you were when the headache struck.

You may determine your headaches are triggered by pollutants – cigarette smoke, for example. If you find yourself returning from work every evening with a headache, it could be due to auto exhaust fumes on the freeway. You may realize you're fine until you have that glass of red wine to relax in the evening. Maybe you have a headache every evening until you've eaten dinner. Low blood sugar could be the culprit in that case.

Sometimes, headaches are a side-effect of medication you are taking for another condition. I took Hismanal for allergies and found that whenever I took it, I'd have severe headaches. I asked the doctor about it, and he pooh-poohed the idea, saying headaches were extremely rare from the medication. I looked the medication up in a reference book (something everyone should have and check before taking any medication) and sure enough, headache was the first side-effect listed. I discontinued the medication and the headaches stopped. Just because something is "rare" doesn't mean it doesn't happen. This time, I was the "rare" one. There's no reason it couldn't be you, too.

Headache is also a sign of overdose on the very painkillers you could be using to stop the pain. If you have to take painkillers frequently, or more than 2 doses a day, it's not a bad idea to do a major reassessment of your headache strategy. The easiest thing to do is to find what triggers the headache and remove the trigger from your life, in the case of offending foods and pollutants. If you have headaches from cigarette smoke, stop smoking and don't hang out with people who do. If you get headaches in the car, keep the windows up and use the air conditioner. If you get a headache when you drink, switch beverages until you find one that allows you to relax, pain-free.

Food can trigger headaches. MSG, a flavor enhancer found commonly in Chinese foods, can trigger migraines. Salad bar items can contain **preservatives** which can trigger migraines in those susceptible. **Caffeine** can sometimes stop a headache, but then again, too much can trigger a headache. Caffeine is also used in some painkillers to boost their effectiveness. People who drink a lot of coffee during the week, but not on weekends, may find they have headaches from caffeine withdrawal. Instead of going cold-turkey, taper off on coffee slowly. Minimize consumption during the week as well.

Don't just think "pain" and reach for the painkillers. Identify the location of the pain. If it's sinus problems, the easiest way to tell is to center the palm of your hand over your nose, so the thumb is on one side, the little finger on the other, the three remaining (hopefully you only have 5 fingers!) along the brow. Lightly tap your fingers to your face. If it hurts, you probably have a sinus headache.

The best thing for sinus problems are decongestants. You may not even be aware that you have congestion. **Decongestants** reduce the swelling and pressure which is what's causing the pain in the first place. Do not take anything containing an antihistamine, as that will only lead to a sinus infection.

While you wait for the decongestants to kick in, you can do something about the pain. **Massaging** the area with something **cold**, reduces swelling and relieves pain. I used a bottle of beer one time as I had no ice, and it worked great! **Warmth** can be helpful as well, as it is relaxing. Try breathing **steam** from a shower or hot water faucet. Do not attempt to breathe steam from a pan of boiling water, you could actually burn yourself. You want warmth and moisture.

If you must take a chemical pain reliever, stay away from acetaminophen (Tylenol). Although it does block the pain, it does nothing to eliminate the cause of the pain. Aspirin or ibuprofen actually reduce swelling. **White willow bark** works like aspirin, in fact it's called "nature's aspirin," and is gentle on the stomach. **Feverfew** is the number one herb in Europe for headache relief. It has been clinically shown to work on migraines. It can cause a drop in blood pressure and diarrhea but has generally been proven safe and effective.

If the source of the pain is towards the base of the skull, it could be due to tension or poor posture. To check, massage the back of your neck, down to your shoulders. If it is sore, you may have found the source of the headache. Take immediate action to improve your posture. You may have pulled something in your neck exercising (sit ups are notorious for this if you use your neck and head to pull yourself up), been carrying something too heavy or awkwardly, or been lifting heavy objects.

The thing to do for this type of pain is first of all, relax. Soak in a hot tub, get someone to give you a massage, lay down for awhile. Usually, you'll find the pain goes away pretty quickly on its own. Once again, **white willow bark** is a good pain reliever for sore muscles, which is what started your problem. A heating pad also works well to relax muscles and relieve the pain. **Valerian** is a safe and effective anti-tension herb.

Another type of headache is the stress headache. It can mimic the tension/muscle headache in that you can feel the pain emanating from the base of the neck between the shoulders, but the actual source is stress and anxiety. Oftentimes, you'll feel pain at the top of the head. The same remedies that work with the tension headache can work for the immediate pain, but you'll be hard-pressed to avoid future headaches without some life -changes.

If your life has been particularly stressful lately due to some ongoing changes you'll have to allow run their course, for example: the death of a loved one, the loss of a job, a move or the breakup of a relationship, you won't be able to do much about the immediate stress you're experiencing. What you can do is change the way you experience the stress. You can acknowledge that you have a lot of stress in your life and find ways to better help you cope and relieve the stress.

Exercise is one of the best all around stress reducers. Not only does exercise release chemicals which bring about a natural high, concentrating on exercise allows you to shelve your anxieties for a time, and take a mental vacation. After exercise, the **endorphins** released into the bloodstream make you feel stronger and better able to handle the tough road ahead.

Herbs can be extremely helpful in dealing with stress. **Valerian** can relieve feelings of anxiety and is one of the best sleep aids. While it is essential you get enough rest when dealing with stress, sleep can be elusive when there is a lot on your mind.

Most herbal remedies for headache, besides feverfew and white willow bark which act on the actual pain, work by facilitating relaxation. **Chamomile tea** is recommended, as is mint tea. **Fresh mint leaves** placed on your forehead will relieve tension.

There are many herbs for headache relief. Skullcap, **wood betony, bayberry, blue vervain, butcher's broom, catnip, dong quai** (for migraines, particularly those related to female cycles), **eyebright, false unicorn, hops, kelp, lady's slipper, lobelia, passion flower, rose hips, sage, yarrow and yerba santa**. Some of these herbs work better than others for headaches. It all depends on what type of headache you have, what the cause is and what you need. You don't have to try all of the herbs, but as some are harder than others to come by, we always like to give you options.

An herbal combination tea for headaches is one prepared with 1/2 teaspoon each of **sage, peppermint, rosemary,** and **hops**. Pour two cups of boiling water over the mixture and let it steep for ten minutes. Add a pinch of ginger and sweeten to taste. All the herbs in this tea are known for their relaxing, calming effects. It is recommended the tea be drunk before bedtime.

Another tea that is good for stress and stress-headaches is **primrose tea**. Pour two cups of boiling water over three teaspoons of dried primrose flowers and leaves. Cover and let stand 15 minutes. Strain and sweeten. Drink warm or hot. This tea is a good antidepressant.

Other herbs for depression and stress are **gotu kola, gingko biloba, cayenne, red clover,** and **catnip,** among many others. Experiment a little. I've found that gotu kola and cayenne work wonders if I'm feeling depressed or stressed. I take cayenne every day and heavy up if I feel life is a strain. Gotu kola pulled me out of depression and made me feel more like myself.

Migraines are a major problem for some people. Many can feel a migraine coming on and notice the first symptom can be nausea. If this is you, treat the nausea first, then the headache. Nausea can be due to too much stomach acid and these gastric juices may hinder the absorption of certain over-the-counter and prescription analgesics, which may make them less effective in relieving the pain of your headache. **Aloe juice** is wonderful at soothing upset stomachs of all kinds. Another benefit is that with aloe, you don't have to worry about any conflicts in medication. If you take a Pepto-Bismal type remedy, you have to be careful as it contains salycylates which can combine negatively if taking a pain reliever with salycylate acid, like aspirin. Too much can lead to ringing in the ears or even internal bleeding.

For some, a sensitivity to light is a symptom of migraine. If light seems to hurt your eyes, don't force yourself to endure the discomfort. Wear dark glasses, or close the blinds. Better yet, take a nap. For many migraine sufferers, sleep is the only thing that interrupts the pain cycle of a migraine.

Feverfew was tested on migraines in Britain with excellent results. You can buy it as tea, in capsule form singly, or as part of an herbal combination formula for migraines. Check your local health store.

Heat seems to help many with migraines. Some people find relief from the blast of hot air from a hair dryer. It's worth a shot. A widely recommended cure calls for boiling a pot of **vinegar and water** and inhaling the fumes for several minutes. At the very least, you'd have clear sinuses.

An herbal remedy you can make at home for migraines is one tablespoon chopped stinking iris to one pint water. Boil gently for 15 minutes. Strain and take up to three tablespoons per day. This also has a slight laxative effect, so don't be alarmed!

Many people who take cayenne have found they get fewer migraines. This would be due in part at least, to cayenne's beneficial effect on the circulatory system.

Migraines and headaches due to hormonal changes or birth control pills are relatively common. If you are taking the pill and notice migraines whether they are new to you or even if they seem to have increased in severity since you started the pill, it's a good idea to consult your doctor about changing the dose. Birth control pills come in a wide array of dosages and types and there is no reason to suffer any side-effects while on them. Other birth control methods which can lead to headaches and migraines are the implant type, where a small implant is inserted under the skin in the upper arm, and Depo Provera, which is given in the form of a shot every three months.

If you aren't on any hormonal birth control method or form of hormonal therapy, yet suffer from migraines and headaches either premenstrually or during menstruation, there are herbs and PMS formulas you can try. Blessed thistle is good for balancing hormones. It also improves the flow of oxygen to the brain and aids in circulation. It is recommended for girls going through puberty and those with menstrual problems. You will find it sold both singly and in combinations with Squawvine (excellent for menstrual and pre-menstrual difficulties), red raspberry leaves (good for morning sickness, menstrual and pre-menstrual problems), cramp bark (stops cramps both during menstruation and ovulation), false unicorn (good for headaches, feminine problems) and uva ursi (healing and soothing to genito-urinary tract) with usually a dash of cayenne, ginger, and goldenseal (a natural antibiotic). passion flower is also recommended for headaches and PMS. Experiment a little. There are many, many herbal combinations for women and many will provide a noticeable difference in how you feel.

A friend swears by the homeopathic PMS formula. I've tried it and don't notice a thing. Yet, I make sure I have Dr. John Christopher's FemMend or Nature's Herbs Blessed Thistle combination or Heartfoods Women's Day formula on hand at all times. Sometimes, I'll combine them. Everyone is different. What works for your unique body chemistry won't necessarily work for your best friend. But usually, something WILL work.

If your headaches are associated with physical exertion, changes in vision, weakness, numbness or paralysis of the limbs, it's time to seek professional advice. See your doctor. If your headaches are not responsive to any attempts you've made to ease them, it would also be a good idea to seek medical assistance. For most of us though, headaches are no more than a pain in the "head," as opposed to a pain in the opposite region! In that case, one of our natural remedies should help.

Keep Those New Years' Resolutions

By Kelly Quinn

Every year, it's the same old story. After a wild holiday season, we look ahead to the new year and resolve to do better, this time. This year, we will lose weight. This year, we won't drink so much. This year, we stop smoking.

January is a big time for those in the health industry. Diet clinics, exercise studios, treatment centers, all do a booming business catering to customers who've decided to make lifestyle changes. Go to any health club in the first week of January and you'll have a hard time even finding a place to park¡the place is packed. Come back the first week in February and you'll be able to park right next to the door.

That's because most resolutions, no matter how sincerely made, almost inevitably get broken. It's not simply a matter of willpower and desire to change, it is also vitally important to have the means to follow through and make changes we can live with.

How many times have you vowed that this is the year you'll lose weight and get in shape, only to spend the first week of your new regimen in pain or eating anything you can get your hands on when the torment of denial fails to make the numbers on the scale smaller or your jeans bigger?

How many times have you sworn off cigarettes or alcohol, only to find yourself losing your mind for want of a smoke or unable to socialize at a party because they all seem to be having a better time than you—because they can suck up the booze and you're stuck with flat Perrier? C'mon, you tell yourself. One drink can't hurt, just to be sociable. The next day after you sleep off yet another hangover, you wonder where you went wrong.

Don't be too hard on yourself. You aren't a weak-willed slug. You just didn't have all the right tools to create the new, improved, you. The purpose of this article is to give you the information you need to make the changes you desire.

WEIGHT LOSS

Let's start with the most common resolution first: losing weight and getting in shape. I write my resolutions down every year so I can see how I did when the year is up. For many, many years, number one on my list was lose weight and get in shape. Finally, after many years of self-loathing and trial and error, I figured it out. Now, my resolution is to maintain my body at its present fitness level. Maintenance is a life-long commitment, but a heck of a lot easier than losing the weight and getting fit in the first place.

So how do you do it? First of all, take a good, hard look at yourself and see what you've got to work with. Anyone 20% over the norm for their age, build and height is considered obese. If you are supposed to weigh 100 lbs. and you weigh 125, you could be considered obese.

Obesity is not fun or healthy. Besides the lack of fashion options, obese people are more likely to have kidney trouble, heart disease, diabetes, high blood pressure and liver damage. A change in eating habits is critically important. Believe it or not, it is possible to be obese, but malnourished at the same time. There is little nutritional content in candy bars or chips.

Exercise is the best way to control weight, not a strict, starvation-level diet. Exercise rids the body of fat and maintains muscle tone. When planning your regimen, remember, carbohydrates and fats—

not proteins—are the main sources of energy used by your muscles. If there are insufficient carbohydrates available for fuel (for example if you've been starving yourself all day but insist on working out anyway), the body will use protein for energy and take it anywhere it can get it. That means you will burn muscle, rather than fat. Protein is also needed for structural repair and to build tissue.

However, your need for protein does not increase with exercise. In fact, excess protein increases the elimination of urine by the body. This can cause dehydration and hinder performance and endurance. Because excess protein is not stored, a strain is put on the liver and kidneys.

So, when planning your diet, you want to be sure to include some protein, but more carbohydrates. It takes carbohydrates to convert fat to energy. When you exercise, you burn fat. You also increase muscle mass. Muscle requires more calories to maintain than fat. This means that a person with more muscle tissue on their body, pound for pound than a person with more fat on their body, will have a higher metabolism and burn more calories even when at rest. That's why you can cut your calories to starvation level and lose less weight than someone who just cuts out dessert and takes a brisk walk daily.

Your body is geared to help you survive, despite yourself. What I mean here is that your body goes into famine mode the minute you stop the food (fuel) from coming in. It burns protein first, saving precious fat stores for last. Not only will you lose muscle-mass and watch those pecs shrivel away to nothing, but your heart is a muscle, too. Imagine what happens when your body has to start cannibalizing itself for fuel if you don't provide enough. Why do you think anorexics frequently die even after they've started boosting their weight?

Anorexics aren't the only ones who have problems. A study revealed that one-third of patients who went on crash diets of 500 calories or less developed gallstones. There have been fatalities linked to the liquid diet plans as well. Drastic, extreme diets do very little to help the dieter achieve a permanent weight loss. Most weight lost during the first two weeks of dieting is actually fluid. As soon as the dieting stops, the weight returns.

No, starvation isn't the answer. A diet rich in complex carbohydrates and low in fat is. Accompanied with an exercise program you can live with. Too many people join a health club, go on every machine and collapse the next day, unable to move. When something is painful, it tends to discourage us from continuing the activity. Start slowly. You can add additional exercise as you get stronger.

Do something you enjoy. When running was so popular a couple years ago, I tried jogging. All I could think of was how I was going to die and hoped to do it at home so no one would see how obese I was in my jogging outfit. I kept at it for about two weeks, and my perseverance still amazes me. Nowadays, I reserve running for escaping life-threatening situations. Fortunately, I don't have too many of those.

But, I walk. I like to walk and always have. Don't force yourself to do something you hate or you're doomed to failure. If you join a gym, check it out first. Try a free workout or two. Most will let you have a trial two week membership. Take them up on it and use it. You may find that you really enjoy the atmosphere and the equipment. You may also find that the equipment is too difficult for your fitness level, or that you hate working out with other people in the room. Best to know for sure how you feel before plunking down any cash.

Think twice before buying expensive exercise equipment, too. Your body doesn't know the difference between walking on a treadmill or going outside for a walk. Nor can it distinguish between an exercycle or a bicycle. Or a stairmaster or a run up a flight of stairs. The idea of exercise is to make your body move. You don't need expensive equipment for that.

If you find you really like the convenience of pulling out a machine to exercise on, without a care for the weather outside or the time of day, consider buying cheap and upgrading as needed. For $19, you can buy a bench for step-aerobics. The top-of-the-line model costs nearly $100. Mine cost $39, two years ago. I use it about twice a week and it works great. If the one you choose doesn't come with a tape, you can rent a few and try them out before making a purchase.

I have a stair-stepper I bought four years ago. It cost under $200 and I loved it, until the cable broke. A new one is only $3, but it's been on order for almost a year now. You can get an el cheapo model for under $30, nowadays. It doesn't have railings, but for the best and most effective workout, you shouldn't use the rails anyway. The cheap model is perfect for a trial run and by the time it breaks, you'll know if you like the results and the activity itself enough to spend bigger bucks on another machine. If you do, make sure you can get parts for it if needed.

There's nothing wrong with even a cheap, kids jump rope. You can jump in areas of limited space and it is a very intense aerobic workout. Try different things before committing yourself to a major expenditure.

Most people who buy exercise machines wind up storing them unused in the closet or garage. Many machines give you more than you really need for health. The weight machines in particular are overkill. They cost a fortune, don't come assembled, take up a lot of space and really don't do anything a good set of free weights can't do.

When exercising, be sure to avoid dehydration. Drink lots of fluids (tepid water is best, it's readily absorbed by the body—cold water can cause cramping) before, during and after exercise. You can lose 25% more fluids in the winter if exercising outdoors due to the cold—simply the act of breathing in and out vigorously can be dehydrating! If you exercise outside in the cold, a face mask will decrease dehydration.

It is recommended in Prescriptives for Nutritional Healing that exercisers avoid bananas, celery, grapes, peaches and shrimp before workouts, especially if you've been sensitive to them in the past. Severe reactions have occurred after exercising.

The book also recommends: a fast once a month to cleanse the body, drinking 6 to 8 glasses of water a day, and eat extra fiber. Don't think chewing gum will aid in keeping you away from the sweets. Chewing gum actually starts the digestive juices flowing and makes you feel hungry sooner than you otherwise would have. It also overworks the digestive system.

Herbs and supplements can be helpful in weight reduction. **Chromium picolinate** promotes lean muscle mass and helps regulate blood sugar. One 250 mg. supplement a day will do the job. Results are slow, but steady. **Guggalo** lowers fat in the body. **Cayenne** can boost the metabolism as much as 25% and gives you energy to exercise. **Chickweed** cleanses the system and maintains the vitamin/mineral level. **Plantain** reduces hunger and hastens weight loss. **Red clover** is a blood cleanser and mildly suppresses the appetite. **Dandelion** reduces fluids and keeps the system regular.

There are some rather unusual diets and techniques that may actually work. Try these for kicks if you're inclined, we can't make any promises! A weight loss diet center in England reported using one part **vegetable oil** to two parts **apple cider vinegar** in massage to rid the body of fat. They actually had positive results! Use **virgin** olive oil for the vegetable oil if you do this—it requires no refrigeration. Knead lightly but firmly over the desired area, at least three times a week for quick results. This is also good for sore and stiff joints.

College students lost up to 15 pounds in less than two weeks consuming only **baby foods**, fiber *(guar gum or glucomannan)* and **spirulina**. No fat, sugar, salt or chemicals was consumed. Add lots of liquids and you have a diet that will produce fast results.

Weight reduction can be improved by use of a combination of the amino acids **L-ornithine** and **L-arginine** enhanced by **L-lysine**. L-ornithine helps release a growth hormone lacking in adults that burns fat and builds muscle. This combination works best if the body is at rest. Never take an amino-acid formula that doesn't contain L-lysine with L-arginine. Without L-lysine, an imbalance could result, possibly causing an outbreak of cold sores or previously dormant herpes.

There is a drug used for weight-loss: Dimitrophinol. This drug is suspected of causing cataracts. No drug works for losing weight or appetite suppression without side-effects, some of which are potentially lethal. Artificial means to lose weight inevitably result in gaining all and more of the weight back, usually within a year. Don't think artificial sweeteners will reduce your cravings for something sweet, either. The American Cancer Society found that people who used artificial sweeteners actually gained weight. The artificial sweeteners appeared to increase appetite. Saccharin has been linked with bladder cancer in males and aspartame (NutriSweet) has been linked to nerve disorders and damage.

SMOKING

If you decide this is your year to quit smoking, you may find you need the section on weight-loss as well. Smoking raises the metabolism and when you quit, even if you don't eat more, you may very well find yourself gaining weight. Exercise will keep your metabolism up. Don't think of smoking as a weight-loss aid, however. It has been shown that smokers fat accumulates in the stomach area. Stress also increases the weight-gain in the stomach area, so if you are a stressed-out smoker, that may explain a pot-belly.

If you smoke, you've heard the statistics. There is absolutely nothing good about smoking. A few additional facts may help you strengthen your resolve.

Tobacco smoke is the cause of one-third of all cancer deaths and one-fourth of all fatal heart attacks in the U.S. alone. Degenerative diseases linked to cigarette smoking are: lung cancer, chronic bronchitis, heart disease, emphysema, cancer of the mouth and throat, cancer of the bowel, angina, diarrhea, heartburn and peptic ulcers. 350,000 Americans die from smoking every year. That's more than the combined deaths from alcohol, illegal drugs, traffic accidents, suicide and homicide. Each cigarette shortens your life by approximately 7 minutes.

Tobacco smoke contains nicotine, carbon monoxide, carcinogens and hydrogen cyanide among other poisons. Women smokers are particularly at risk. They reach menopause earlier when smoking because chemicals in the tobacco affect the hormone-producing cells in the ovaries. Women smokers face a greater risk of osteoporosis, a higher risk of lung cancer and a much higher risk of cancer of the cervix or uterus.

Men who've smoked for years are much more likely to have abnormally low penile blood pressure, which contributes to the inability to have an erection.

Tobacco can affect the way your body handles prescription and non-prescription drugs. Theodur, for example, must be given in higher doses to smokers. Smoking is also contraindicated in patients taking ulcer medications like Tagamet, Zantac and Pepcid. Birth control pills and other hormone-based contraceptives should never be used by smokers due to the increased risk of strokes and heart attacks.

Quitting smoking is not easy. The physical addiction to nicotine has been likened to that of heroin. Withdrawal symptoms can include: irritability, depression, anxiousness, a phlegmy cough, stomach cramps and headaches. These symptoms usually last no more than a few weeks. The urge to smoke usually passes in 3 to 5 minutes, so you can wait it out.

So how does one quit? The nicotine patch can be helpful to some people. It's a patch that is usually worn on the upper arm which delivers nicotine that is absorbed into the bloodstream. The idea is that if you can get the nicotine from another source, you'll be able to wean yourself off the emotional aspects of the habit, then by gradually reducing the dosage in the patch, wean yourself from the physical addiction. The problems with the patch are two-fold. The first is that unless there is some sort of behavior-modification introduced, the emotional aspects of the habit will be hard to break. The rate of success for the patch is no higher than for those who quit smoking without it.

Another problem is the physical side-effects of the patch itself. Nausea, rashes and dizziness are among the more common reactions. Others include headaches and even heart-attacks. This is because the amount of nicotine delivered may be much higher than your body is used to, if you smoke lower nicotine cigarettes or smoke infrequently. If you wear the patch and sneak a cigarette, the effects can be extremely toxic, even fatal.

You don't have to go the patch route to quit, however. There are many natural ways to enable you to quit smoking. Herbs used to quit smoking include **lobelia, hops, skullcap, cayenne, and valerian.** Some people discover an aversion to smoking after taking cayenne which helps them avoid lapsing into old habits.

A quit smoking formula from the *Pocket Reference Guide* by Debra Nuzzi includes many herbs beneficial to those trying to quit smoking. You can follow her formula and take the herbs all at the same time, or you can try various herbs based on availability. The formula combines herbs to alleviate the nervousness associated with nicotine withdrawal while stimulating detoxification and expectoration.

Anise seed – an anti-spasmodic and expectorant.

Chamomile flower – a sedative, anti-gas, anti-spasmodic herb which also relieves pain.

Dandelion root/leaf – a blood cleanser, stimulates the flow of bile. Lowers cholesterol and blood pressure.

Grindelia buds/flowers – an expectorant, anti-spasmodic, used for bronchitis, sinus congestion.

Licorice root – an expectorant, anti-inflammatory herb.

Lobelia herb – a respiratory stimulant, anti-asthmatic herb used in bronchitis and asthma treatment. Lobelia is similar in composition to tobacco in that it can fool your body into thinking it's had tobacco when it hasn't, yet it doesn't have the averse side-effects including death that tobacco has.

Oat seed – an anti-spasmodic, soothes and supports the nervous system. Helpful in decreasing the irritability associated with nicotine withdrawal.

Valerian root – a powerful nervine used for tension, anxiety, emotional stress and breaking addictions.

Peppermint oil on the tongue can help break the smoking habit and desire. Fresh **carrot juice** is said to be the best preventative against lung cancer. Drink it daily. Tobacco smokers need more **vitamin C** than non-smokers. Brushing your teeth when you feel the urge to smoke can help squelch the desire. You'll also have the whitest teeth in town!

Whatever method you choose to stop smoking, tailor it to your needs. A study found that people who gradually taper off by cutting down on cigarettes smoked daily had the same success rates as those who quit cold turkey. Another thing to remember when you feel you'll lose your mind is that the first three days are supposed to be the worst in quitting. That's because it takes three days for your body to detoxify from your last cigarette. Taking **cayenne pepper** can help speed the detoxifying process.

ALCOHOL

So you've already quit smoking, you're slim and trim and the next thing you want to tackle is alcohol consumption. Alcohol is increasingly unpopular today as more is discovered linking it to birth defects, liver damage, brain damage, pancreatic ills, ulcers, and damage to the central nervous system. Alcohol is actually a human-specific poison. It causes metabolic damage to every cell and depresses the immune system.

Alcohol is particularly hazardous to the unborn and causes birth abnormalities in infants. Alcohol passes through the placenta and into the fetus's bloodstream. The baby's liver must then attempt to metabolize the alcohol, which is not fully developed. If the liver is not developed enough to metabolize the alcohol, the alcohol remains in the infant's system. Growth may be retarded or stunted. The brain may be small and there may be mental retardation. Limbs, joints, fingers and face may be deformed. Heart and kidney defects may occur. Even moderate amounts of alcohol may be harmful, particularly in the first three to four months of pregnancy. Pregnant women should avoid all alcohol.

Alcohol also affects the way your body handles prescription and non-prescription drugs. People on the ulcer medications Tagamet, Zantac and Pepcid should not drink alcohol. Tagamet makes your liver unable to metabolize the booze so you get drunk sooner and stay drunk longer. Cold medications should never be taken with alcohol, nor should allergy medications. Alcohol and aspirin or ibuprofen can lead to stomach bleeding. Alcohol and acetaminophen (Tylenol) can cause liver and kidney damage. Many anti-biotics' effectiveness is inhibited by alcohol. Always ask about mixing booze with any medication, even vitamins.

Alcoholics are often malnourished. Liver damage inhibits the production of digestive enzymes, impairing the body's ability to absorb proteins and fats. The ability to absorb vitamins A, D, E and K is impaired. Liver damage also leads to the retention of fluid, which is why alcoholics may appear overweight and bloated. Alcohol literally kills both liver cells and brain cells.

It takes six hours for each drink to be metabolized and leave your system. Nothing speeds up the process. Coffee results in a wide-awake drunk. Cold showers result in a cold, wet drunk. A woman's menstrual cycle will also affect the way she metabolizes alcohol. Some times of the month tolerance is extremely low.

The body eventually builds a dependence upon the alcohol with continued, heavy drinking. Withdrawal from alcohol is usually most difficult during the first week of abstinence, with physical symptoms of insomnia, rapid pulse, acute anxiety, extreme perspiration, fever, even visual and auditory hallucinations and convulsions may occur with severe alcoholism. If you are an acute alcoholic, medical supervision during detoxification or "drying out" is recommended.

Herbs to ease the process include: **passion flower, lobelia, skullcap,** and **valerian** to relieve tension and anxiety. **Cayenne, alfalfa, chaparral, dandelion, garlic, ginseng, kelp, gotu kola, red clover,** and **yellow dock** aid in the detoxification process and rebuild the body. **Silymarin** *(milk thistle extract)* helps rebuild the liver.

It is best to stay away from drugs and chemical tranquilizers while trying to overcome a dependence on alcohol, as it is easy to replace one addiction with another. None of the herbs for detoxification or relaxation are addictive.

It is important to get proper rest and nutrition to enable the body to repair damage and regain strength. Exercise speeds the elimination of toxins and helps break the dependency on alcohol by relieving stress. It may also help to join a group like Alcoholics Anonymous or one of the many other groups available for those wishing to stop substance abuse. Look in the front of your phone book for hotline numbers and referral services.

Consider restructuring your social life. If every weekend is spent in bars or with people to whom alcohol consumption is a major part of their entertainment activities, if will undoubtedly be more difficult to abstain. Try some new activities where alcohol is not an integral part. You'll have a good time and wake up the next day feeling good, rather than hungover.

Good luck on keeping your New Year's resolutions.

*H*ELP *Y*OURSELF *U*NDERSTAND *H*OMEOPATHY

By Kelly Quinn

*I*t's cropping up more and more in different places: homeopathic medicine. Even some mainstream drugstores now carry homeopathic medicines for PMS, allergies, and other common ailments. What is homeopathic medicine anyway, and does it work?

Homeopathic medicine is a natural medical science that uses naturally occurring substances of plant, mineral, or animal origin, which when taken in very small doses stimulate the body's natural defenses or innate healing powers. The medicines are individually chosen for their ability to cause symptoms similar to those a person is experiencing. The name comes from the Greek: "homoios" means similar and "pathos" means disease or suffering.

The idea is that the body knows what it's doing when trying to combat illnesses. Rather then blocking the symptoms of a cold, for example, the homeopath would use something that in large doses causes similar symptoms. This aids the body in its effort to defend and ultimately cure itself.

The homeopathic concept of "like cures like" is not as unusual as you might think. Conventional medicine uses variations of homeopathic treatment in immunizations and allergy treatments, two of a limited number of treatments in conventional medicine which stimulate the body's own healing processes.

Immunizations and allergy shots are not homeopathy, since homeopathic medicines are more individually prescribed and are given in smaller, safer doses. Homeopathic medicines are used to both treat and prevent disease.

Self-treating with homeopathy can be hit or miss. A homeopathic physician interviews patients in great detail to discover the totality of physical, emotional, and mental symptoms the patient is experiencing. Then the homeopath attempts to find a substance that would cause similar symptoms the person has and gives it in small, specially prepared doses.

For example, the homeopath may prescribe a preparation made from an onion for a person with a burning, watery, nasal discharge and frequent sneezing because onion is also known to cause such symptoms. If the patient has differing symptoms, the medication will not work, but it will not cause side-effects either. If the medicine is the right one, the person will quickly notice an obvious improvement in his condition. Not only do homeopaths find that the medicines help to relieve acute and chronic symptoms, they also strengthen the body so it is less likely the symptoms will return as often or with as much intensity. The same cannot be said for Nyquil!

Conventional treatments for common colds primarily attempt to dry mucus membranes. Homeopaths claim such treatment suppresses the natural defenses of the body, thereby creating side-effects.

Homeopathy is called "alternative medicine" in this country, but it is an integral part of European mainstream medicine. According to a survey in the British Medical Journal, 42% of British physicians refer patients to homeopathic physicians. Homeopathy is even more popular in India, where there are over 100 four-year and five-year homeopathic medical colleges. Homeopathic medicines are regulated by the FDA and are considered over-the-counter drugs. This recognizes them as basically safe and allows them to be sold without a doctor's prescription. A bit of trivia: the FDA was in part created by a homeopathic physician, Dr. Royal Copeland in the late 1930's.

The way homeopathic medicines are made makes them quite different from any other type of medicine, including herbal medicine. They are manufactured through a procedure called "potentization" which is a process of diluting and shaking, again and again. For example, a tincture of Belladonna would be diluted with nine parts or even ninety-nine parts distilled water. It's shaken vigorously and then diluted again, one part of the mixture to nine or ninety-nine parts distilled water. The process of diluting and shaking is continued anywhere from one to over a million times. By the time the medicine is ready, it is almost impossible to detect the active ingredient.

Homeopaths have discovered the more a medicine in potentized (diluted), the longer it acts, the deeper it acts and the fewer doses are generally needed.

Homeopathic medicines are usually taken more frequently than conventional medicines while symptoms are present. For example, for a hacking cough, you may find you are directed to take four tiny pills (or drops) every hour symptoms are present, then once or twice a day until the illness is gone.

The fact that homeopaths use such small doses has caused some to wonder if the medicines are real or simply act as a placebo. There is much historical, clinical, and scientific evidence to show that the medicines work, regardless of whether a person believes in homeopathy or not.

Why such small doses? The key in homeopathy is finding the correct medicine for each individual. This is why self-treatment can be hit or miss. Fortunately, there are no side-effects and homeopathic medicines are relatively cheap (especially when compared with traditional medicines), so you can afford to experiment a little in finding the correct medication for you. If it's the wrong one, you simply won't feel any better. Try again.

How do I treat myself? Traditionally, homeopaths prescribe an individualized medicine based on the patient's unique pattern of symptoms. However, homeopaths have been using formulas for years. A formula combines two to eight homeopathic medicines that are all known to be effective in treating a specific condition.

A formula allows one product to serve a larger number of people and makes homeopathic medicine more readily available. Also, some formulas may have a broader effect in treating people suffering from a specific condition than an individual medicine. Just as herbalists will combine various herbs in a formula and find they act synergistically to increase the therapeutic benefits, homeopathic formulas can have similar action.

That's why if you walk into a health-food store that carries homeopathic remedies, you'll see formulas for an assortment of illnesses lining the shelves. In many stores, you can also buy a single ingredient remedy, usually by matching your specific symptoms with a list in a book the store has for that use. When using single-ingredient formulas, it is crucial to be specific and clear about the symptoms. If the product is for someone else, a child for instance, it can be difficult. I tried to buy a remedy for my daughter, who had complained of an earache, but the book listed symptoms in such minute detail that I had to give up and go with a formula for a wider variety of symptoms.

Some formulas work better than others. The remedies by Medicine From Nature, where most of the information on homeopathy was gathered from this story, never seem to quite work on me. My friend, however, takes them and has nothing but praise for them and their quick results. I've had better luck with the Hyland's brand of homeopathic medicines. I particularly like their cold and cough line. They have many more formulas for allergies and colds. What's great about homeopathy is if the medicine doesn't work pretty quickly, you can try a different formula without having to wait 6 to 12 hours for the medication to entirely leave your system, as you do with conventional medicines.

Even though homeopathic formulas make it easier for homeopathy to reach more people and allow patients to better treat themselves, the power of individually chosen single homeopathic medicine should not be underestimated. The correctly chosen homeopathic medicine can effectively heal a person's chronic or even hereditary condition. Although formulas may temporarily relieve a chronic condition, they rarely cure it. The correct medicine can also raise the patient's general level of health, so the person is more resistant to physical and psychological ailments, acute and chronic.

If homeopathy is so great, why doesn't my doctor use it? At the turn of the century, 15% of American doctors were homeopathic physicians. There were 22 homeopathic medical schools (including Boston University, University of Michigan, New York Medical College, University of Minnesota, and Hahnemann Medical College) and over 1,000 homeopathic pharmacies.

Despite the incredible popularity of homeopathy just 90 years ago, it has sharply declined due to strident attacks from the American Medical Association. Still, homeopathy has persisted and has recently experienced a tremendous resurgence of interest. New research confirming the effectiveness of the homeopathic medicines has brought increased media attention and greater scientific respectability to the field. Numerous training and educational programs have sprung up helping to create more professional homeopaths.

More educated consumers is a goal of those involved in homeopathy, both physicians and the manufacturers of homeopathic products. A free booklet, sponsored by Medicine From Nature, called *A Beginner's Guide To Homeopathy* was used as a major source for this article. There are many other books available on the subject of homeopathy, but you'll find the free booklet a nice thing to have on hand as it explains homeopathy in an easy-to-understand manner, and the price is right. Check your local health store.

Don't be afraid to experiment with homeopathic products. Amazingly, they *do* work—in most cases anyway. The cough formula from Hyland's works better than any cough syrup or whole herb formula I've ever tried. The only annoyance with homeopathic remedies is that you need frequent doses, often within a half hour before eating or drinking anything. You may have to take a formula every hour when symptoms are severe, three or four times a day after that.

When you're ill, it's very easy to over-medicate or incorrectly treat your symptoms, often leading to more serious illness. Someone with a simple cold, for example, will take antihistamines and cough suppressants and wind up with a sinus infection and bronchitis. There is no danger of that happening with homeopathic medicines, as they do not suppress the symptoms. They work with the body, enabling it to heal itself.

Let people call homeopathy "alternative medicine." Alternatives are a good thing to have. More alternatives mean more choices. More choices means better health care.

─────────────── ❧ ───────────────

HELP YOURSELF HEAL A WOUND

By Kelly Quinn

My daughter, Heather, somehow managed to remove a huge chunk of skin from her shin. It was more than your average scrape and by the time she told me, it was already a couple of days old.

It still hadn't gotten a scab on it and it bled through her sock, through the makeshift bandages she'd applied. The risk of infection increases with every minute the wound is open. It was imperative we keep the wound clean and dry and some sort of scab form to prevent infection.

But what do you do when the wound doesn't take care of all that by itself? Usually you hardly notice a cut or scrape, other than to give it a quick wash before forgetting all about it. Nature takes care of the rest. The scab is nature's Band-Aid. On occasion, you get a wound that doesn't follow nature's plan. It stays open and you have to step in.

When you get a break in the skin, the first thing to do is think CLEAN. The injury must be cleaned, the area around it cleaned, to prevent more germs from entering the body at the wound-site. Soap and warm water are usually enough to clean a wound and the area around it. Bleeding usually cleanses the inside of the wound itself by washing out any germs and debris that entered the body with the break in the skin.

Don't use alcohol to clean the wound. *Avoid* peroxide and mercurochrome to sanitize wounds. All hurt like the dickens and really don't do any better at cleaning the site than good old soap and water. They can even be detrimental to tissue. Don't scrub the wound either, unless it's absolutely necessary. Rinsing and patting are the way to go. The tissue is already traumatized, you don't want to make it worse.

The next treatment to emphasize is dry. Until the wound is DRY, really dry, leave it alone. Sit back and relax a few minutes, tell the tale of your misfortune to anyone around and let the wound dry. You can pat it *gently* with a clean, dry towel, but if it hurts to do that, don't bother. Let the air get at it.

When the wound is dry and the bleeding has stopped, very often you're done. Most wounds *do not* require a bandage. We've become a Band-Aid-happy country over the years, what with the proliferation of those keen adhesive strips. But for the most part, Band-Aids do more harm than good and interfere with nature taking its course.

Your body is smart, you see. The bleeding cleanses the wound, the clotting stops the blood after the wound has been cleansed, the scab that forms is nature's Band-Aid and protects the wound from further damage allowing it to heal. The pain and bruising from a wound are your body's way of telling you where the trauma is and to protect the area. And don't panic if you see a clear fluid oozing out of the wound. This is not a sign of infection, but rather an antibody-containing fluid. Clever, huh?

When you slap on a bandage, usually it's coated in plastic, is barely big enough to cover the wound and goes on too tightly. No air can get in. With the warmth and perspiration of your body, the wound becomes moist. Bacteria find an ideal environment in which to grow. And it grows, quickly. By the time you peek under the Band-Aid again, you often notice the wound has become infected. Sometimes we even help it along by coating the wound with a sticky cream to "promote healing."

Basically, the only time you need a bandage is if the wound is in a place where it could be easily reopened or bumped. If you think you have to hold the skin together with a bandage to promote healing, you don't need a bandage, you need stitches.

Before you dress the wound, avoid putting anything on it that will keep it wet. Creams and antibiotic salves should be used rarely, if at all. If you have a wound that seems to be getting too dry as it heals and there is danger of the wound reopening, a small amount of a cream or ointment can be helpful.

So what do you put on the wound? Usually, nothing. Sometimes, some type of protection is a good idea, particularly when the wound doesn't appear to be closing well. In that case, you know you'll likely have an open wound for awhile and it's important to use something to speed healing.

Cayenne red pepper works phenomenally well on wounds and cuts of all types. It stops infection, makes a nice hard protective crust over the wound and starts healing. The big fear in using red pepper is that it may sting. That depends on the wound, but it actually stings for several seconds and then kills the pain and soreness. Cayenne has been used with tremendous success on canker sores and cold sores as well, and treatment is not overly painful. My son had a scrape on his hand that became infected and tried cayenne. Yes, it did hurt for a few seconds, but it healed it so well that now he automatically reaches for the cayenne if he gets a wound. The crust it formed stayed put until the wound was completely healed, even through showering and swimming.

If you are dealing with someone who is afraid of cayenne's sting, or maybe *you* are, **aloe vera** is very healing for all types of wounds, including burns and sunburn. Use it right from the plant, or buy it in gel form or juice.

Comfrey is a major ingredient in many healing creams available at health stores.

Garlic kills germs and speeds healing. You can open a garlic capsule and spread the liquid on the wound. If all you have is powdered garlic, go ahead and put some of that on the cut. Yes, you can use fresh garlic. Peel and bruise a bulb and rub the juice on the wound. It may sting.

Slippery elm is soothing and promotes healing. You can make a poultice with it and apply it that way, or any way you can get it to sit on the wound. It will not harm the surrounding tissues and doesn't sting.

Echinacea kills germs and speeds healing. You can use it in extract form, as a poultice, even make a tea and dab it on the wound with a cotton ball.

St. John's wort can be used in a poultice to promote healing.

White oak bark works well in a poultice.

Plantain is very soothing to the damaged area and speeds healing. If you can only find the leaves, you can place one of them over the injured area and loosely cover it with a bandage. Otherwise, use it in a poultice.

Chaparral disinfects and speeds healing. Make a poultice or dab on strong tea with a cotton ball at regular intervals.

Other herbs that promote healing are: **bayberry, bistort, burock, camomile, chickweed, dandelion, goldenseal, horseradish, horsetail, lobelia, myrrh, papaya** (you can just dab on a little meat tenderizer if it contains papain which is from papaya or even place a thin slice of fresh papaya over the wound and secure loosely with a bandage), **peach bark, sage, taheebo, valerian, willow, witch hazel, wood betony, yarrow, and yucca.**

All the above herbs work well in poultices. A *poultice* is a moist, hot herb pack applied locally. If the herb is fresh, crush and bruise it. Powdered herb should be mixed with water or other liquid to form a paste. Spread on a clean cloth and cover the affected area. Leave on for several hours. Always use a fresh poultice, they should never be reused.

Don't be afraid to experiment. Maybe you don't want to, or for some reason can't make a poultice. Try a strong tea, dabbed on with a cotton ball. Try making a paste of the herb with warm water and slapping it on the affected area.

You can also use these herbs to make an Antiseptic Spray Formula, according to Debra Nuzzi in the *Pocket Herbal Reference Guide:*

Calendula flower: anti-inflammatory, astringent, styptic, antifungal, topically for wounds, ulcers, burns, abscesses.

Cayenne: antiseptic, styptic.

Chaparral: antibiotic, anti-viral, antiseptic, specific for infections.
Echinacea: antiseptic, anti-microbial, anti-viral, stimulates immune response.
Goldenseal: antiseptic, used topically for infection, sore throat, ulceration. **Caution:** do not apply fresh Goldenseal directly to skin, it can cause blistering and pain.
Myrrh: used externally on cuts and abrasions, forms natural Band-Aid. Antiseptic, anti-microbial, astringent. Used for mouth ulcers, sore throats, gingivitis, pyorrhea.
Eucalyptus oil: antiseptic, bactericide, disinfectant.

You can use all, some, or even just one, of these herbs at a time to make an antiseptic spray. First, make a tea with the herbs. Strain off herbs, Put liquid in a spray bottle, and va! You have your own version of Bactine, except yours works better and costs a heck of a lot less!

What if you are totally out of every herb imaginable, or you're away from home and need a quick fix? Try sugar or honey. Both speed healing and fight infection.

What if the bleeding just won't stop on it's own? First, raise the affected area above your heart if at all possible. Put gentle but firm pressure on the area right above the wound. Do not use a tourniquet, as you could cut off too much of the blood supply.

There are herbs that stop bleeding almost instantly. It's a good idea to have at least one of these on hand at all times, in case of emergencies. **Goldenseal** and **Plantain** applied directly to the wound stop bleeding, as does **Cayenne**. A bit more about the pain factor of cayenne here: I've spoken to many people who tell me of times they've had serious bleeding they've stopped cold with cayenne. All tell me it did not hurt. It's been speculated that cayenne shorts out the nerve that carries the "pain" signal within seconds of application. Cayenne is actually used as an anesthetic. It's not unusual for an anesthetic to sting for a second before the pain stops altogether. If the wound is one like a scrape, it will probably sting a bit more as there is more surface area of the skin exposed.

Cool water can often slow or stop bleeding if it is not too severe. If bleeding is severe, use what herbs you have to stop bleeding, at the same time applying pressure. It's a good idea to call 911 or seek immediate professional assistance if bleeding is heavy and hard to stop, as the patient may have severed an artery or other important blood system. A transfusion may be required.

How do you know if a cut necessitates stitches? Many facial

wounds require stitches to ensure they heal with a minimum of scarring. If the cut is very deep, you may need stitches. If the cut is wider than a quarter inch or too raged to close evenly, you may want to see a doctor. When the injury occurs in an area of tendons or nerves or you see anything sticking out of the wound, see a doctor! If you can't feel the area that has been injured and can't move it, see a doctor!

Another type of wound that is treated a bit differently than a cut is a burn. Put the burned area under *cool,* **not cold** *water.* The cool water will actually remove some of the heat of the burn. Cold water will further damage already damaged tissues.

Forget the myth about putting butter on a burn. Butter or other oily substances will merely seal in the heat and lead to more damage. Keep a cool cloth on the burn until the pain is gone. Apply aloe vera on the burn when the heat is gone and take it internally. Take vitamin C hourly to prevent infection and speed healing. Honey speeds healing and prevents infection, so does sugar. Vitamin E spread on the burn accelerates healing. Use a capsule you've cut open and spread the fluid on the burn. A slice of potato placed on the burn (raw, of course!) will help draw the heat out of the affected area. A coating of milk can relieve pain from a mild burn or sunburn.

Let's get back to Heather's wound and what we did for it. By the time she showed it to me, it was well on its way to becoming infected. I rummaged around and found some samples I'd picked up at a health convention. They were extracts to be taken internally. The directions on each vial suggested we put the contents into a beverage. Each was the perfect size for a one-time application to her wound.

We got rid of the Band-Aids she had covering the wound. She carefully cleansed it, let it air dry, then put a capsule of powdered garlic on the wound. Then she went to bed, with no covering on the injury so it could get air.

The next day, it already looked much better, it had managed to develop a scab. She put a sample of echinacea extract on it, covered it with a loose bandage, just enough to protect against it being bumped, and went to school.

That night, after her shower, she once again let the injury air-dry, then put a sample of aloe gel on it before retiring. I noticed she no longer cringed with trepidation that someone would inadvertently bump her injury. She was back to wrestling with the dog and being a regular kid.

What a difference a couple of days of the proper treatment makes! The wound has scabbed over nicely, she no longer favors the injured leg and soon will be left with little more than a memory of her injury.

And the confidence that comes from knowing how to take better care of herself.

January 1994

Dear Reader,

Now that it's a new year, many of us are giving our bodies a once-over and taking stock of the results of too much holiday indulgence. Even if we were the souls of restraint over the holidays, it's more than likely we've added a few pounds in the past couple of months.

Winter is tough on a body, both physically and emotionally. The cooler weather and lack of sunlight tend to put us in hibernation-mode. It's been shown that the metabolism has a tendency to slow in winter, perhaps as a way of preparing us for famine. Historically, food used to be hard to come by in the winter months, fresh vegetables and fruits next to impossible until spring. Nowadays, of course, the problem isn't too little food, it's too much; although fresh fruits and vegetables can be expensive and lacking in variety.

To give your vegetable consumption a boost, consider adding fresh fruit and vegetable juice to your diet. You couldn't pay me to eat a carrot/apple/broccoli puree, but I just drank a glass of juice in which I threw in those same ingredients. It tasted great and was so filling that I skipped dessert. You don't need anything too fancy, even a $30 juicer works. If you are going to be getting into juicing in a big way, you may want to consider one of the pricier models which get more juice from the whole fruit or vegetable. You may even want to pick up a book on juicing. Some claim it can cure you of whatever ails you. I never noticed any big difference medicinally, but I do know it's a great way to up your intake of beta-carotene.

Start slowly, though. If you find yourself drinking huge vats of carrot juice, you could find you start to take on an orange hue. It's not dangerous, just a little disconcerting. Also, when I try something, I tend to go overboard. When I started juicing, I would drink three 16 ounce glasses of juice a day and started to get stomachaches.

When I cut my consumption by half, my stomach felt fine.

A lot of people feel depressed in the winter. Cabin-fever can be a real problem when you're trapped inside all the time. Seasonal depression or seasonal affective disorder (SAD) is now recognized by the American Psychiatric Association as a psychiatric syndrome. The disorder is characterized by social isolation, depression, withdrawal, a craving for carbohydrates, weight gain, loss of energy, tendency to sleep longer, and a decreased sex drive. If this sounds like you, the solution can be a simple one: get outside.

When I lived in Wisconsin where the winters are long and cold, every February I'd feel like I was ready to lose my mind. I'd fantasize about running away and joining the Coast Guard, anything to change what I perceived as a hellish existence. Later on, I realized the problem wasn't my life, it was me! I had many of the symptoms of SAD. It wasn't until I moved to a place where I could go outside without fear of freezing to death that I made my discovery. One year, February passed and I didn't "go nuts." I felt fine. I realized after reading about SAD that I'd gotten through the winter without a hitch because I'd been outside a lot more and had gotten more sunlight.

Humans need sunlight. If you live somewhere where you really can't get outside, or it's cloudy for days on end, consider investing in some bright lights. Stay in a brightly lit environment for 45 minutes to an hour a day. If the sun comes out, plant yourself in a sunbeam, even if you just sit there and read. Exercise helps fight depression of course, but the key in fighting SAD is to expose yourself to as much light as possible. You'll be amazed at the difference in how you feel!

Take care of yourself,

Kelly Quinn

*A*ROMATHERAPY AND *E*SSENTIAL *O*ILS

By Kelly Quinn

While doing research for an article on herbs for women, I noticed aromatherapy cropped up in my reference materials with increasing frequency. I'd never really paid much attention to the concept before, other than in using aromatherapy candles for congestion when my children had colds. They always worked really well, but I'd never really pursued the topic in any depth.

Until now, that is. It's a lot more complicated than just smelling things. You can't really do anything in aromatherapy without also learning about essential oils.

Essential oils are the essences of plants. They are used in making perfumes, cooking, aromatherapy, and even orally. Since the focus of this piece is aromatherapy, we're not going to do more than lightly touch upon any uses of essential oils, except in aromatherapy applications. Remember however, that many of the oils can be taken orally or used topically and are very similar to herbal extracts in their healing and soothing properties.

First of all, what exactly is aromatherapy? In answering that question, I learned that the human sense of smell is 10,000 times as powerful as the sense of taste. Yet, it is the least utilized of the senses. Aromatherapy has been used since ancient times and is experiencing a resurgence today. Fragrance is a type of healing that operates on physical, emotional and spiritual levels. It stimulates and calms, alters mental states, boosts the immune system, relieves pain and balances bodily functions.

Essential oils are used in aromatherapy. They are the hormones of plants, the concentrated active ingredients of herbs. They are generally steam-distilled from a wide range of flowers, roots, leaves, barks and resins or cold pressed from the rinds of citrus fruits. Only natural essential herbs are healers. The oils you'd buy in a grocery store are mostly water and alcohol, containing very little of the essence of the plant you're trying to use. They are merely flavoring agents.

Essential oils are more than flavoring agents or perfumes, however. Depending on the essence you choose, they can be germicidal and anti-viral, anti-depressants, aphrodisiacs, hormonal balancers, detoxificants, anticarcinogenics, mental stimulants, fever and blood pressure reducers and more.

They can have a profound effect that goes beyond cognitive knowledge or memory, even supposedly on cellular levels. Different fragrances do different things and have different healing attributes. Scents may be used singly or in combinations. They can be diluted or placed directly on the skin, used in massage oils or baths, added to creams or lotions, used in a steam vaporizer, sprayed in the air, put on light bulbs or in candle lamps to heat, or just sniffed from the bottle.

Some essential oils are very expensive. They can range in price from about $3.00 to hundreds of dollars, for a very small bottle. Happily, they are usually used by the drop and keep indefinitely. They should be stored in amber glass to keep them safe from the degenerative effects of heat, light and air.

To achieve any benefits, the oils must be natural oils and absolutely pure. Because they are so concentrated and therefore, extremely potent, essential oils should always be kept out of the reach of children. Always dilute essential oils in vegetable oil when applying near the eyes, mouth, nose or genitals.

There are some oils that are unsafe for internal use: Balsalm Peru, Camphor, Cedarwood, Cypress, Fir Needle, Frankincense, Myrrh, Patchouli, Pennyroyal, Vetiver and Wintergreen.

Avoid these oils if epileptic: Fennel, Sage, Rosemary and Hyssop.

Avoid these during pregnancy, both internally and externally: Pennyroyal, Anise, Basil, Clary Sage, Sweet Fennel, Hyssop, Juniper, Marjoram, Myrrh, Peppermint, Rosemary, Sage and Wintergreen.

The following can irritate skin (use sparingly): Lemon, Lime, Orange, Tangerine, Bergamot (stay out of direct sunlight after application), Basil, Black Pepper, Cinnamon, Cassia, Citronella, Clove Bud, Fir Needle, Ginger, Lemongrass, Nutmeg, Thyme or large amounts of Cinnamon Leaf or Peppermint.

It's easier than it looks to use essential oils. To try them in a massage oil, blend 1-3% essential oils with vegetable oils like sweet almond, grapeseed, or apricot kernel oil. Try some in your bath, a drop on a light bulb or in a sachet.

Some of the main essential oils and their uses are:
Anise: stimulates circulation and respiration.
Basil: clarifies mental faculties, inhale aroma to lift fatigue.
Bergamot: used to treat depression.
Camphor: stimulant.
Cedarwood: stimulant.
3HAMOMILE: calming, refreshing, relieves stress, irritability, depression, migraines and digestive problems. Aids in restful sleep.
Cinnamon: stimulating effect on body, aphrodisiac.
Cypress: a few drops on pillow are good for colds and flu.
Eucalyptus: good for congestion, nasal and chest.
Fennel: digestive aid.
Germanium: sedative, fights anxiety.
Ginger: stimulant, aphrodisiac.
Juniper Berry: diuretic, eliminates toxins, speeds digestion, fights kidney and bladder disorders.
Lavender: relaxes both nervous system and muscular system, calming effect.
Marjoram: sedative, also good in massage oil for sensitive skin and face.
Melissa: antidepressant.
Myrrh: add to massage oil to rejuvenate skin.
Nutmeg: stimulant.
Orange: lifts mood, fights fatigue and depression.
Patchouli: relaxing, aphrodisiac.
Pennyroyal: stimulant, relieves seasickness. **Warning:** abortive.
Black Pepper: stimulates digestion.
Peppermint: stimulant.
Petitgrain: sedative.
Rose: relieves anxiety, depression, circulatory problems.
Rosemary: improves memory, mental acuity.
Clary Sage: relaxant.
Sandalwood: relaxant, aphrodisiac.
Spearmint: stimulating to mind and body.
Tangerine: energizing, antidepressant.
Thyme: energizing physically and mentally.
Wintergreen: stimulant, may relieve headache.

Ylang Ylang: euphoric effect, emotionally soothing, strong aphrodisical properties, attracts opposite sex.

You'll find some of these oils harder to get than others. I looked for Ylang Ylang at three different stores, before finally finding it as an ingredient in a massage oil.

Candles are another option in aromatherapy. There are candles for congestion, headaches, relaxation, even some reputed to aid in weight loss. At the very least, they can lend a nice ambiance to a room with very little effort.

Aromatherapy can be a fun, relatively cheap form of therapy to experiment with. Like many therapies, some things will work better for you than others. I'd suggest picking a few of the more readily available essential oils and experimenting with them as oils or candles and see what happens. That's what I intend to do.

WOMEN: HELP YOURSELF FEEL GREAT! (PART I)

By Kelly Quinn

It's wonderful to be a woman, but sometimes, it isn't easy. Women suffer many maladies and discomforts uniquely female. Menstruation, pre-menstrual syndrome, pregnancy, menopause, breast abnormalities, even chronic fatigue syndrome are female-specific disruptions which can have far-reaching effects on our lives.

Women often get short-shrift when it comes to health care. For one thing, as the "nurturers," we rarely get a chance to nurture ourselves. It certainly doesn't help that the medical establishment is for the most part male-dominated. Medical tests and studies are routinely done on men, rarely are women included in the testing or the results. So, frequently, when women are treated by conventional medicine for any physical problem, they are being treated as if they were male. While many drugs and therapies work equally well on both sexes, many differ in their efficacy.

There is no denying that women are physically different than men. Even herbs sometimes work differently on women. Some herbs are uniquely male herbs, some female, and some should not be taken by nursing or pregnant women. Most importantly, if you can match the condition you want to treat with the right herbs and supplements, you can often alleviate or even cure the affliction, safely and naturally. The herbs and supplements listed in the following article are safe and effective. I've tried many of them myself and enthusiastically testify to their efficacy.

Women have different nutritional needs than men. Menstruation, ovulation, pregnancy, breast feeding and menopause all add different nutritional requirements. Using the Recommended Daily Allowance (RDA, or the new RDI) to determine the complete nutritional needs of women virtually guarantees a woman will be deficient in some vitamins or minerals at varying times of the month. The following are some recommended supplements women should have on hand to replenish the nutritional balance of the body, both during "special times" and every day.

BEE POLLEN

Bee pollen is a whole food remedy. It boosts the immune system, is a major remedy for allergies, sinusitis, hay fever or asthma and will reduce symptoms of those ailments. Bee pollen boosts endurance, retards aging and speeds healing. It is a brain stimulant, alleviates menstrual problems and promotes orgasm by balancing the reproductive system's hormones. Bee pollen helps pregnancy and milk production, and reduces the symptoms of menopause. It may prevent or delay the appearance of malignant breast tumors and reduce existing ones. The recommended dose is two tablets or an ounce of bee pollen a day. It doesn't have to be local pollen, although it is recommended local pollen be used if combating allergy symptoms. If using pollen to fight allergies, be aware of your symptoms. Some people experience a worsening of symptoms after initial use. If that is the case, decrease dosage and build a tolerance slowly. Other bee products have similar benefits and work equally well: try **propolis, honey, royal jelly** and **honeycomb**. Bee pollen may increase the appetite slightly.

GARLIC

Garlic is antibacterial, antiviral, antifungal. It boosts the immune system, lowers high blood pressure, and is particularly important in healing systemic candida albicans, vaginal yeast infections and recurrent bladder infections. To stop candida or yeast infections, take 2 tablets three times a day until symptoms stop, then decrease the dose. Stay on a program of maintenance of two tablets daily for at least three months more, increasing dose at the first signs of colds, infections or illnesses. Garlic is essential for women with herpes.

APPLE CIDER VINEGAR

Apple cider vinegar replenishes minerals and potassium in the body. Useful in treating osteoarthritis, apple cider vinegar is also a preventative against osteoporosis. Used for digestive upsets, food poisoning (prevents and remedies), kidney and bladder infections, chronic fatigue, headaches, dizziness, high blood pressure, sinusitis, allergies and infertility. Apple cider vinegar is antibacterial, antifungal, and boosts the immune system. Don't substitute white vinegar, they aren't the same. For daily use, mix with honey if desired and drink 1 teaspoonful apple cider vinegar in a glass of water alone or with meals. For chronic diseases use the mixture one to three times a day. For acute illnesses, use as needed. For sore throats, try 1 teaspoonful of apple cider vinegar in a glass of water and gargle as needed.

For specific complaints, the following natural remedies can be of tremendous value in eliminating or controlling the condition. All are non-toxic and can be added to whatever therapy you're currently using without negative effects.

BACKACHES

Half of all women experience back trouble within their lives and one in ten lives with chronic back pain. High heels, carrying small (and not so small) children and child-related paraphernalia, pregnancy and stress all play a role in backaches. Back pain can also be a symptom of pelvic, kidney or bladder problems, gall stones and gynecological disorders.

For relief of pain, try **feverfew, white willow bark, skullcap,** valerian and hops. You can make a tea of **skullcap, valerian** and **catnip**. It's best to drink the tea before going to bed as the herbs work as a muscle relaxant and you're likely to feel drowsy.

For relief of recurring backaches, try **horsetail grass**, an herb that aids in calcium uptake. **Alfalfa** is an important blood cleanser and provides the body with crucial nutrients.

Breast Lumps

Remember: when discovering a lump in the breast, not all lumps are indicative of cancer. Cysts and fibrocystic breast conditions are common in women. Avoiding caffeine is usually extremely helpful. You can also make a tea with one ounce of **red clover** and one ounce **blue violet leaf** to a pint of water. This will cleanse the system and dissolve most breast lumps as well as uterine and ovarian fibroids.

Candida Albicans

Candida can affect many parts of the body. It can show up as mouth or foot thrush, skin rashes, vaginal infections, chronic fatigue syndrome, hypoglycemia, arthritis, sinusitis, digestive upsets, abdominal pain, PMS, depression, constipation and diarrhea. Many more women than men are affected by candida. Women who are diabetic or pregnant, have been taking antibiotics, or contraceptive pills, are undergoing chemotherapy or taking steroids are at greater risk. Women with compromised immune systems are also more prone to developing candida albicans.

The source of the candida imbalance is intestinal. The natural balance of bacteria in the digestive system is easily disrupted by hormones, antibiotics or an excess of refined carbohydrates. Once entrenched, candida is difficult to diagnose due to the plethora of symptoms and even more difficult to treat.

Drugs for yeast infections, i.e. Nystatin, Monostat, Nyzoral and Amphotericin B, depress the immune system and develop drug resistant yeast/candida strains. Holistic healing focuses on diet, immune system strengthening, replenishing the levels of "good" bacteria and eliminating yeast by detoxification.

To control and eliminate candida, it is important to eat as natural a diet as possible, restricting sugars, refined carbohydrates, yeasts and preservatives. Eat **acidophilus** as frequently as possible either in yogurt with active cultures or as supplements.

Herbs that eliminate candida albicans are: **Pau d'arco, black walnut, white oak bark, buchu,** and **chaparral,** which also aid in rebuilding the immune system. Try alternating **pau d'arco** and **clove** teas. To sweeten your tea (or anything else, for that matter), try stevia. It's sweeter than sugar and does not encourage the growth of yeast.

Garlic is crucial in the treatment of candida. Take two tablets or capsules, three times a day. If you notice flu-like symptoms, a general feeling of malaise, a whitish coating on the tongue, discolored stools, constipation or diarrhea after a couple of days on the garlic, be encouraged. These are signs the yeast is dying and is being eliminated from the body. If any of these encouraging signs get too uncomfortable, decrease the dosage (don't stop the treatment!) for a few days, then increase it again. The symptoms generally end after about a week. Take the garlic for at least three months longer, decreasing gradually to one to two tablets or capsules a day.

CHRONIC FATIGUE SYNDROME

Three times more women than men are afflicted with chronic fatigue syndrome. The symptoms include extreme exhaustion, flu-like symptoms, swollen glands, recurrent colds, intestinal problems, anxiety, depression, irritability and mood swings, aching muscles and joints, headaches, memory and concentration loss. Prolonged symptoms result in immune system burn-out, endocrine and adrenal exhaustion. Persistent symptoms for longer than six months and an elevated antibody count are the basis for diagnosing chronic fatigue. Chronic fatigue can result from a number of ailments other than the Epstein Barr virus.

Proper nutrition is extremely important in fighting chronic fatigue. Increase your intake of **vitamin** C and add a good quality **multivitamin** tablet. Sixty percent of chronic fatigue can be traced to candida albicans, so it's a good idea to take acidophilus to return the bacterial balance to the intestines.

Herbs are frequently used to treat chronic fatigue with excellent results. **Cayenne** is a potent antiviral and antibacterial agent. It protects against secondary infections, builds the immune system and gradually inactivates the Epstein Barr virus. Take it before eating.

Pau d'arco, **chaparral** and **burdock** are used to cleanse and detoxify the system. All balance the immune system. **Red clover** and **aloe vera juice** can be extremely helpful as well.

An old home remedy for chronic fatigue which has shown positive results in a European study is a **cool bath**. The water should be about 60 to 65 degrees Fahrenheit, and the patient soaks for approximately ten minutes. Don't let the water get too cold. The idea is that cooling the body may kill the virus. More studies are underway.

Cystitis (*Bladder Infections*):

Thirty times more women than men experience urinary tract infections and 4% suffer chronically. Many bladder infections are caused by an imbalance of intestinal flora, the after-effect of taking antibiotics or other drugs. Cystitis is also linked to systemic candida albicans. Birth control pills are a factor, along with poorly fitting diaphragms, allergies to spermicides and liver problems.

Caffeine and alcohol can be irritants as can frequent sexual activity. Not consuming enough water can exacerbate the condition as can tight-fitting nylon underwear or pantyhose.

It is important to drink lots of water to keep the bacteria diluted and flush out the bladder. Urinating before and after intercourse flushes the harmful bacteria from the area. Wiping from front to back, rather than back to front after going to the bathroom will also cut the risk of cystitis.

The symptoms of a bladder infection include frequent urination, often with burning or pain. Frequently, you'll feel the urge to urinate immediately after emptying your bladder, or feel the urge to go, but nothing's there. There may be pain or cramping in the urethra. The urine may have a strong smell, look cloudy or contain blood. The abdomen may appear or feel bloated.

Untreated bladder infections can spread to the kidneys which can be serious. If you experience pain at the back or at waist level, the kidneys are most likely involved.

In fighting cystitis, it is important to take 1000 mg. **vitamin C** every hour. **Acidophilus** is important if you're on antibiotics. **Cranberry juice** acidifies the urine and kills bacteria, as does **cherry juice, lemon juice, buttermilk** or 2 tbsp. **apple cider vinegar** in a glass of water.

Herbs for bladder infections include: **Juniper berries, buchu, cornsilk, marshmallow root, nettles, parsley, dandelion,** and **uva ursi** to soothe and cleanse. Herbal antibiotics recommended for cystitis are **goldenseal, echinacea** or **pau d'arco.**

Depression

There are many causes of depression, both physical and emotional. For all types, try increasing your intake of **B-complex vitamins.**

Women who are on the pill or notice the depression is related to the menstrual cycle need **vitamin B6** (250-500 mg. per day) and **folic acid** (400 mcg. daily). **Lecithin** is important for brain and nerve function, but not for use by manic-depressives. Vitamin C is important to fight stress, 1000-3000 mg. daily.

Herbs which fight stress and ease depression include: **passion flower, skullcap, catnip,** or **chamomile**. Herbs which fight lethargy include: **gotu kola, damiana, lavender, rosemary, peppermint, cloves, borage** and **cayenne**. Try the herbs separately, or mix your own combination. Most of them make a nice tea. **Black cohosh** balances hormones, particularly in women over the age of 40.

HERPES

There are three main types of herpes: cold sores on the lips, genital herpes and herpes zoster (shingles), the same virus that causes chicken pox. Herpes is incurable. The virus may lay dormant for long periods of time, flaring up when under stress or if the immune system is compromised.

Genital herpes afflicts over 35% of American women. Most new cases are in white women between 20-40 years old. The first attack is usually the worst, most often occurring within three weeks of exposure. New outbreaks usually stop after menopause.

The infection is contagious during outbreaks, when blisters or open sores are present. If a pregnant woman has herpes, a cesarean section may be necessary to protect the infant if active sores are present at the time of delivery.

Beta-carotene prevents the infection from worsening. **Vitamin C** with **bioflavonoids**, 1000-5000 mg. a day strengthens the immune system. **Vitamin E** (400-800 I.U. a day) speeds healing and can be used topically on the sores.

Herbs are very beneficial in the treatment of herpes. Topically, they soothe and speed healing. Try **licorice root gel, echinacea, butternut, comfrey** and **goldenseal** made into a paste with water, **black walnut** or **slippery elm**. **Aloe vera gel, calendula** and **myrrh** mixed with **witch hazel** also soothe and relieve discomfort.

Internally, try **burdock root tea, red clover, sassafras, chaparral, white oak, pau d'arco, echinacea, Oregon grape root** and **goldenseal**. They are blood cleansing herbs and natural antibiotics.

There are home remedies you may already have in the cupboard which can be of help in treating herpes. **Lemon juice** applied to tingling areas will reduce blister formation and duration. **Garlic** is said to cure herpes and prevent future outbreaks. Try 12 capsules daily, then three every four hours while awake for three days. This will not stop an attack already in progress, but should shorten the duration and the severity.

MENOPAUSE

Although a natural part of a woman's life, menopause is frequently treated as a disease. The insistence on treating menopause as an illness has led to a booming business in estrogen replacement therapy. Estrogen replacement increases cancer of the uterus and breast from 5 to 12 times average. Estrogen also causes water retention, increases asthma severity, heart disease, kidney stones, epilepsy, migraines and the incidence of stroke. Holistic remedies are a safe and effective way of dealing with the discomforts of menopause.

Vitamin E, along with a **B-complex vitamin**, is the remedy of choice for hot flashes and all menopausal symptoms, including emotional. Use it topically for vaginal dryness. Internally start with 400 I.U. daily, increasing weekly by 100 I.U. until the dosage is 800 to 1600 I.U., divided into several doses a day. Stop at the dose that ends hot flashes.

For hot flashes, add **vitamin C**, at 3000 mg. minimum dose. **Calcium/magnesium** (up to 2000 mg. calcium/1000 mg. magnesium) eases emotional symptoms and is essential to prevent bone loss.

Evening primrose oil and **black currant oil** act as a sedative and diuretic and also ease hot flashes. They are important for estrogen production. **Germanium** will also help menopausal symptoms, use 60 mg. two times daily.

Dong quai is primary in treating the symptoms of menopause. Try it in tablets or tinctures (a few drops under the tongue will stop a hot flash in progress). It gives energy, lowers high blood pressure, treats profuse menses and vaginal dryness. While dong quai is an estrogen balancer, it is not an estrogen itself. Some women may experience a feeling of nervousness while taking the herb. If so, switch to **black cohosh**, which has similar effects but is a progesterone balancing herb.

False unicorn root, licorice root, damiana, mistletoe, gotu kola, motherwort, sage, passion flower, **lady's slipper, chaste tree** (vitex), **oats** and **squawvine** are herbs for menopause. Try **red raspberry** as a relaxant. **Angelica, false unicorn, dong quai, wild yam** or **licorice root** are estrogen herbs. Licorice can raise blood pressure, so avoid it if you suffer from hypertension.

Sarsaparilla is a progesterone balancer which is helpful to many women. **Lady's slipper** is for anxiety and insomnia, **false unicorn** helps menopause related depression, and **passion flower** calms the mind and the body. **Shepherd's purse** or **nettles**, especially if used with **alfalfa**, lessens heavy flows and breakthrough bleeding. **Motherwort** is helpful in easing early discomforts of menopause, regulating erratic cycles, easing heavy or clotted flows, irritability and hot flashes.

MENSTRUATION AND CHILDBIRTH

Medical drugs for menstruation discomforts add toxins and sometimes hormones which worsen any imbalances in the body. The drugs increase symptoms or have side-effects that can be worse than the symptoms being treated, all without fixing the cause of the problems. Holistic healing reaches the sources of the distress working with women's bodies, rather than blocking symptoms and aggravating the problem.

Overall nutrition is important. A complete **calcium/magnesium** supplement that contains 1000-2000 mg. of calcium and half that amount of magnesium can help ease menstrual difficulties immensely. This can be taken in three to four doses a day. Take with water or water with a teaspoon **apple cider vinegar** for better absorption. This can be taken hourly to relieve acute cramps or pains.

For many women, this is enough to stop cramps. For more relief, try a **B-complex** vitamin of 50-100 mg. three times a day. This is especially important for women on the pill, or those who smoke. Women on the pill who experience tension, bloating, acne or anxiety need extra B_6 of 50-400 mg. a day. Vitamins B_5 and B_{12} are stress and fatigue reducers. 1000-3000 mg. of **vitamin C** with **bioflavonoids** can help reduce heavy flows. 400 I.U. **vitamin D** daily will assist in calcium absorption. Cravings for chocolate, sugar or salt signify a deficiency of **calcium**, **magnesium** or **zinc**.

For breast tenderness, or if you smoke or are on the pill, it's recommended you take 400-800 I.U. **vitamin E**, or 25,000 I.U. daily of **beta carotene**.

For menstrual-related headaches and to balance hormones, try **evening primrose** or **black currant oil, lecithin,** and/or **manganese**. **Chromium** can also help stabilize hormonal balance.

It's wise to take your extra vitamins and supplements daily (not just when menstruating), then increase the amounts of calcium/

magnesium and B-complex vitamins in the last three to eight days before the flow begins, with smaller amounts during the rest of the month.

Herbs have made the difference between having to spend the first couple days of my period curled up in bed with a heating pad and whimpering in pain, to being completely surprised at the onset of my period. I take low dosages of these herbs most of the month, increasing when I get my period. I no longer suffer from PMS or need an extra set of clothing for the first few days of my cycle.

Dong quai can be the answer to PMS, cramping, bloating, vaginal dryness, fibroids, heavy bleeding, irregular cycles and depression. Start the herb slowly, stop if symptoms increase rather than decreasing.

Black cohosh is useful for ovarian cramps and pain. Blue cohosh or raspberry leaf fight PMS and cramping. Red raspberry also reduces menstrual flow.

Motherwort is a menstrual balancer, both for lack of periods and for pre-menopausal women. It also helps pelvic inflammation when combined with echinacea or goldenseal.

Use crampbark, wild yam, blue cohosh or squawvine for difficult periods. For heavy or painful periods, try crampbark, red raspberry, strawberry leaf or white oak bark. Sarsaparilla is a hormone-balancing herb.

For pain or tension, take valerian, skullcap, hops, passion flower, feverfew or cramp bark. Raspberry leaf is good for pregnancy, false unicorn root can prevent a threatened miscarriage.

Shepherd's purse and nettles can control heavy bleeding or hemorrhage. They are also used after childbirth.

To bring on menstruation, try basil, catnip, angelica, parsley, black cohosh, rosemary or ginger. Siberian ginseng is used for PMS and for menopause, but is not for use by hypoglycemicsdong quai is recommended. Motherwort, raspberry leaf, dong quai, wild yam, rosemary, black cohosh and blue cohosh regulate cycles. Use blue cohosh in women under 40, black cohosh for women over 40.

For nausea with periods, use peppermint or peppermint with chamomile in a tea. Pennyroyal increases blood flow, as does blazing star, feverfew, squawvine or tansy. Parsley, nettles, squawvine, dandelion, or blue cohosh reduce water retention.

OSTEOPOROSIS

Seventy percent of osteoporosis sufferers are women. It afflicts one-quarter of all women past menopause. Estrogen deficiency, lack of calcium, prolonged stress, smoking, alcohol, many childbirth's, fluoridated or soft water, thyroid or parathyroid imbalance, birth control pills and vitamin/mineral deficiencies have all been found to be causes of the ailment. Some drugs, including antibiotics, steroids, anti-inflammatories (ibuprofen, for example), surgical gastrectomies and overuse of bicarbonate of soda (baking soda), may be other causes.

The medical establishment's solution of estrogen replacement therapy to prevent osteoporosis puts the patient at greater risk of cancer. When minerals are deficient, the body draws them from the bones, causing bone weakening and thinning. Symptoms of osteoporosis include back pain, loss of height, spinal curvatures, pain on bearing weight, muscle spasms and spontaneous fractures in the hips, lower back, legs or vertebrae, usually in women over 50. Women who are vegetarians are at less risk, with an average bone loss of 7%, compared to 35% for meat eaters.

The bone thinning of osteoporosis is not apparent until it's too late. It doesn't show on X-rays until 30% of the bone mass has been lost. Many times, the first sign of the ailment is a broken bone.

Women of fair complexion, thin and small-boned, have gone through a natural early menopause, have never been pregnant, have a family history of the disease, smoke, live sedentary lifestyles, drink alcohol, soft drinks or caffeine to excess, use cortisone, anticoagulants or anti-seizure drugs long-term, have liver or kidney disease, overactive endocrine glands, digestive disorders or have had their ovaries removed are at even greater risk for osteoporosis. Even drinking water is suspectfluoride leaches calcium from the bones.

The need for **calcium** increases with age. Use 1000-2000 mg. calcium daily, with half that amount of **magnesium. Vitamin C** should be increased to 1000-3000 mg. a day for younger women, 3000 mg. a day for women over 40. Vitamin C deficiency has been linked to osteoporosis. If you have bone pain or already have osteoporosis, try **germanium**. This will prevent new fractures and lessen pain.

Herbs most helpful in preventing and treating osteoporosis include **alfalfa**, which contains all vitamins and minerals and enhances assimilation. **Horsetail grass** or **oatstraw** are high in calcium. **Feverfew** contains minerals and vitamins, reduces pain, menopausal symptoms and migraines. **Nettles** and **comfrey** are high in minerals.

It's important to eat lots of leafy green vegetables and vegetable proteins. Drink spring water rather than fluoridated tap water or distilled water which has been stripped of minerals your body needs.

I've tried many of these supplements and herbs to remedy discomforts and generally improve my overall health and well-being with dramatic success.

March 1994

Dear Reader,

Now that you know the best herbs for men, herbs for better sex, and part two of the herbs for women, there are many ways to take charge of your physical and emotional health, even save your life.

I've had some time to experiment on myself with some of the herbs mentioned in the women's herbs article and the herbs for sex article. Experimenting is always fun, and I've discovered some herbs which I've added to my daily regimen.

Damiana is in both the women's herbs story and recommended as an herb to improve your sex life. I've been taking it for a couple of months and noticed more of a general feeling of well-being. I feel my body is perhaps more in balance, hormonally at least.

Siberian Ginseng is something I started after doing the article on herbs for sex. It figures pretty heavily in recommended herbs for both men and women. I noticed a definite increase in energy. I also sick in over a year, but I finally caught a cold in February. It only lasted four days, and I was functional throughout. I did notice I had to watch how much I take of the Siberian Ginseng—if I'm going to have a regular day, and take more than two in the morning it can make me feel wired. If I'm going out, I'll take two or three in the evening.

Bee pollen is a big player for women. I've been taking it for a few months now and can't say I've noticed much of anything, either positive or negative. But as a natural food supplement, I'll probably keep taking it.

I also tried some essential oils. I can't say aromatherapy has made me a believer. While the oils smelled nice, I didn't notice enough of a difference from the many cheaper massage oils on the market that simply smell good.

I did have a positive experience with an herb I'd like to pass along. I had been fighting off a chest cold and didn't want to take an expectorant because most commercial expectorants just make me tired. I found a bottle of a Pleurisy Root combination and took five capsules. Within a half hour, I realized I wasn't feeling the urge to cough as frequently and my chest was much clearer. Included in the combination were: ephedra, pleurisy root, wild cherry bark, slippery elm bark, plantain, mullein leaves, chickweed, horehound, licorice root, ginger root and saw palmetto berries. This combination could make you feel a little wired if you took too much, if that happens, taper off the dosage. I plan to take a few whenever I notice chest congestion.

Hopefully, the results of some of my recent experimentation can help you take better care of yourself.

Kelly Quinn

P.S. As always, everyone is different. What didn't work for me may very well work for you. By the same token, what works for me may not work for you. Experiment and <u>Help Yourself to Health</u>!

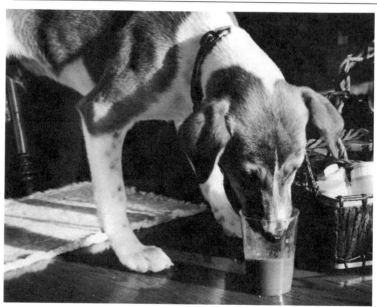

Bailey the beagle likes his dragon cocktails with cayenne and a touch of garlic.

Help Yourself Choose the Right Herbs for Men

By Kelly Quinn

*U*nlike modern medicine, herbs are for the most part unisex in their efficacy and usefulness. Most of the medications used in conventional medicine are tested on men and prescribed based on the results of those tests.

Herbs, on the other hand, have been used for thousands of years on both sexes. The information pertaining to usage and dosage is based on the experience of both men and women.

There are certain ailments that are primarily male, just as there are problems that are uniquely female. Herbs for those gender-specific ailments can make all the difference in a man's ability to maintain optimum health, both physically and emotionally.

HYPERTENSION

Garlic lowers high blood pressure and raises low blood pressure. Also, try **cayenne, crampbark, yarrow, onion, hawthorn berries, siberian ginseng** or **vervain**.

It is important in treating hypertension to limit the amount of sodium in the diet, while increasing the intake of potassium. Focus on lots of fresh fruit and vegetables, plaintain, dandelion and kelp, all of which are high in potassium.

Avoid fats in your diet and lose weight if you're overweight. Obesity is directly linked to high blood pressure, cholesterol and excessive secretion of insulin which can lead to diabetes.

Exercise frequently. This not only helps rid your body of excess weight, it lowers blood pressure all by itself, even if there are no changes in diet or weight.

Limit alcohol, stop smoking and cut down on caffeine, all of which raise blood pressure.

ARTERIOSCLEROSIS

Garlic, the wonder-herb to the rescue! Three cloves of garlic a day will cut cholesterol build-up in half. Also try **hawthorn, linden,** ginkgo biloba, yarrow and cayenne.

Diet is important. Avoid lots of meat, egg, dairy, salt and excess oils. A diet high in vegetables, fruits and complex carbohydrates is important. Avoid alcohol and if you smoke, stop.

Stress: Long term unabated stress tends to have a "grinding down" effect, usually culminating in illness. There are said to be three phases to an individual's reaction to stress:

1. *Alarm Phase:* in which one experiences an intitial adrenaline rush reaction. The classic "fight or flight" response.
2. *Resistance Phase:* in which the body recovers to a level superior to the pre-stress state. This includes adrenal, liver and nervous system responses.
3. *Exhaustion Phase:* in which there can be a depletion and breakdown of any recovery demonstrated in the Resistance Phase due to continuing exposure to the source of stress.

To deal with stress, try nervine relaxants **black cohosh, cramp-bark, chamomile, skullcap** and **lavender** to help soften the physical reactions to anxiety.

To allow you to get the rest you need, try **valerian, passion flower, vervain, hops, catnip, lemon balm, chamomile** and **red clover.**

If stress is upsetting your stomach, try **chamomile, lemon balm, peppermint, wild yam, fennel** and **marshmallow.**

If stress is affecting your heart and/or circulatory system, take **hawthorn, ginkgo biloba, cayenne, motherwort** and **linden blossoms.**

If stress and anxiety leave you short of breath, try **gumweed, wild cherry bark, lobelia** or **wild lettuce.**

If you're in a long-term stressful situation, you will likely find the effects of continuous anxiety and tension result in some ancillary physical and psychological problems. Try to match one of the following herbs with your condition:

St. John's wort: is a nervine with anti-inflammatory and sedative properties.

Vervain: is a nervine tonic which is also antispasmodic and hepatic.

Damiana: is a nervine which is a urinary antiseptic and laxative.

For example, if you have frequent headaches and can't relax, St. John's Wort would be a logical first choice. If your muscles are tense in reaction to stress, Vervain may be the herb for you. If stress makes it difficult to enjoy your "daily constitutional," Damiana would be a good herb to try.

If depression occurs as the result of long-term stress, use St. John's wort, damiana, lavender or lemon balm to lift depression.

Long-term stress can depress the immune system, leading to illness. To boost immune response, take astragalus, echinacea, pau d'arco, cayenne and myrrh. Siberian ginseng, licorice or suma support the adrenal glands as well as the overall immune system.

ULCERS

Ulcers can be stress related. Whether ulcers are gastric or duodenal, it is important to eat a low-fiber diet during the acute phase of the illness. Reduce your intake of protein as it is the most difficult for the stomach to process. Once the symptoms are reduced, proteins and fiber can be gradually reintroduced.

Herbs to soothe and heal ulcers include **marshmallow root, comfrey root** and **slippery elm bark. Goldenseal** heals the mucus membranes. **Agrimony, American cranesbill, bayberry or meadowsweet strengthen the tissue and helps stop the ulcers from bleeding. Meadowsweet** lso settles the stomach and reduces the impact of overacidity.

Hops, valerian or chamomile will aid digestion and help ease stress and nervousness which contribute to and aggravate ulcers.

Cayenne, believe it or not, is used successfully to heal ulcers and stop internal bleeding.

BENIGN PROSTATIC ENLARGEMENT (BHP):

A common problem affecting men later in life, the enlargement of the prostate causes pain and difficulty in urinating. The condition occurs in approximately 50% to 60% of men between the ages of 40-59 years. The condition has a tendency to be progressive, but it is not always.

There seem to be three stages of prostatic enlargement. In the first stage, the stream of urine grows thinner and the urge to urinate increases. Some men notice it takes longer to begin urination. This stage is very responsive to herbal treatment.

In the second stage, retention of urine increases and the bladder never fully empties, leaving residual urine.

In the third stage, the residual urine increases, stagnates and distends the bladder, causing back pressure and eventually kidney damage and uremia. Surgical intervention is necessary at this point.

Herbs to take, particularly in the first stage are: saw palmetto, sarsaparilla, Siberian ginseng, marshmallow root, echinacea and Oregon grape root.

PROSTITIS

Is an inflammation or infection of the prostate gland. This can inflame the prostatic urethra and ultimately the bladder. The symptoms of prostitis are characterized by: an aching pain in the area of the prostate, pain on sitting, leaking urine, difficult urination, difficulty emptying the bladder, sometimes blood in the urine and often chills and fever. Prostitis is often caused by stress, excesses in diet (especially over-consumption of caffeine and alcohol), lack of exercise, or as a secondary infection.

Discomfort can be alleviated by using a firm seat, the avoidance of cold, damp, long sittings, avoiding alcohol, caffeine, cooked hot spices and sexual excess. The urge to urinate must be attended to immediately, as the bladder must not be permitted to be over-distended. Extreme difficulty in urination may be relieved by sitting in a tub of warm water to urinate. Drink lots of water to flush the system and dilute the urine.

Treatment includes:
1. Relax. Use stress management techniques, exercise and herbs like valerian, cramp bark and skullcap help relax muscles.
2. Drink lots of water.
3. Eat lightly, foods that are easy to digest.
4. Throughout the day, eat up to 1/2 cup of **pumpkin seeds**. This respirates the internal organs, decongests the prostate gland and lessens residual urine. Also heavy up on **poppy seeds, sunflower seeds** and **sesame seeds.**
5. Take 800 I.U. of **vitamin E** daily, 400-600 mg. **calcium/magnesium,** and **zinc picolinate** or **amino chelated zinc** 20-50 mg.
6. Apply hot and cold packs to the prostate area. Apply hot and cold in a ratio of 4 to 1. This means 4-8 minutes of heat, followed by 1-2 minutes of cold. Do this 2-3 times a session, two times a day or more. This reduces inflammation.

7. Herbs to try:
- Male reproductive system tonics: **saw palmetto**, **Siberian ginseng, suma**.
- Genito-urinary system tonics and astringents to strengthen and heal: yarrow, **horsetail**, **buchu**, **candelion**.
- Diuretics to prevent excess buildup of urine: **hydrangea**, **couch grass**, cleavers, cornsilk, **watermelon seed**.
- Immune System Enhancers: **echinacea, astragalus, Siberian ginseng**.
- Urinary system anti-microbials to prevent infection: Oregon grape, **echinacea, uva ursi, couch grass, saw palmetto**.
- Demulcents to soothe and protect urinary system: couch grass, cornsilk, marshmallow, comfrey.

Hopefully, through the use of herbs and common sense treatments, you'll be able to avoid many of the side-effects and discomforts which afflict men, especially during middle age and beyond.

WOMEN:
HELP YOURSELF
FEEL GREAT! (Part II)

By Kelly Quinn

We offer herbal and natural remedies for the uniquely female problems like Menstruation, Migraines, Nursing, Osteoporosis, and Pregnancy.

MENSTRUATION

Medical drugs for menstruation discomforts add toxins and sometimes hormones which worsen any imbalances in the body. The drugs increase symptoms or have side-effects that can be worse than the symptoms being treated, all without fixing the cause of the problems. Holistic healing reaches the sources of the distress working with women's bodies, rather than blocking symptoms and aggravating the problem.

Overall nutrition is important. A complete **calcium/magnesium** supplement that contains 1000-2000 mg. of calcium and half that amount of magnesium can help ease menstrual difficulties immensely. This can be taken in three to four doses a day. Take with water or water with a **teaspoon apple cider vinegar** for better absorption. This can be taken hourly to relieve acute cramps or pains.

For many women, this is enough to stop cramps. For more relief, take a **B-complex vitamin** of 50-100 mg. three times a day. This is especially important for women on the pill, or those who smoke. Women on the pill who experience tension, bloating, acne or anxiety need extra B_6 of 50-400 mg. a day. Vitamins B_5 and B_{12} are stress and fatigue reducers. A 1000-3000 mg. of **vitamin C with bioflavinoids** can help reduce heavy flows. A 400 I.U. **vitamin D** daily will assist in calcium absorption. Cravings for chocolate, sugar or salt signify a deficiency of calcium, magnesium or zinc.

For breast tenderness, or if you smoke or are on the pill, it's recommended you take 400-800 I.U. **vitamin E**, or 25,000 I.U. daily of **beta carotene**.

For menstrual-related headaches and to balance hormones, take **evening primrose** or **black currant oil**, **lecithin**, or/and **manganese**. **Chromium** can also help stabilize hormonal balance.

It's wise to take your extra vitamins and supplements daily (not just when menstruating), then increase the amounts of calcium/magnesium and B-complex vitamins in the last three to eight days before the flow begins, with smaller amounts during the rest of the month.

Herbs have made the difference between having to spend the first couple days of my period curled up in bed with a heating pad and whimpering in pain, to being completely surprised at the onset of my period. I take low dosages of these herbs most of the month, increasing when I get my period. I no longer suffer from PMS or need an extra set of clothing for the first few days of my cycle.

Dong quai can be the answer to PMS, cramping, bloating, vaginal dryness, fibroids, heavy bleeding, irregular cycles and depression. Start the herb slowly, stop if symptoms increase rather than decreasing.

Black cohosh is useful for ovarian cramps and pain. Blue cohosh or raspberry leaf fight PMS and cramping. Red raspberry also reduces menstrual flow.

Motherwort is a menstrual balancer, both for lack of periods and for pre-menopausal women. It also helps pelvic inflammation when combined with echinacea or goldenseal.

Use crampbark, wild yam, blue cohosh or squawvine for difficult periods. For heavy or painful periods, try crampbark, red raspberry, strawberry leaf or white oak bark. Sarsaparilla is a hormone-balancing herb.

For pain or tension, take valerian, skullcap, hops, passion flower, feverfew or cramp bark. Raspberry leaf is good for pregnancy, false unicorn root can prevent a threatened miscarriage.

Shepherd's purse and nettles can control heavy bleeding or hemorrhage. They are also used after childbirth.

To bring on menstruation, try basil, catnip, angelica, parsley, black cohosh, rosemary or ginger. Siberian ginseng is used for PMS and for menopause, but is not for use by hypoglycemics—dong quai is recommended. Motherwort, raspberry leaf, dong quai, wild yam, rosemary, black cohosh and blue cohosh regulate cycles. Use blue cohosh in women under 40, black cohosh for women over 40.

For nausea with periods, use peppermint or peppermint with chamomile in a tea. Pennyroyal increases blood flow, as does blazing star, feverfew, squawvine or tansy. Parsley, nettles, squawvine, dandelion, or blue cohosh reduce water retention.

MIGRAINES

Migraines are a major problem for many women. They can be due to many causes: allergies, stress, food sensitivities and hormonal changes. Nausea is often the first symptom of a migraine. In this case, take care of the nausea first as it usually indicates excess stomach acid, which can hinder the absorption of any pain reliever for the migraine itself. Aloe juice is great at soothing upset stomachs of all kinds. With aloe, you needn't worry about conflicting medication.

Sensitivity to light can also indicate a migraine. If light bothers you, don't force yourself to endure the discomfort. Wear dark glasses, close the blinds, take a nap. For many migraine sufferers, sleep is the best cure for an impending migraine.

There are many herbs which can stop a migraine in progress, prevent recurrence, and alleviate the condition which may lead to the migraine in the first place. **Feverfew** works well on migraines. You can buy it in tea, in capsule form, or as part of an herbal combination formula for migraines.

Another cure for a migraine in progress calls for boiling a pot of **vinegar** and water and inhaling the fumes for several minutes. An herbal remedy you can make at home is one tablespoon chopped **stinking iris** to one pint water. Boil gently for 15 minutes. Strain and take up to three tablespoons per day. This has a slight laxative effect.

People who take **cayenne** often find they get fewer migraines. This would be due at least in part to cayenne's beneficial effect on the circulatory system.

Migraines due to hormonal changes or birth control pills are common. If you are taking the pill and have migraines, see your doctor. In fact, if you are on any form of hormonally-based birth control, see your doctor if you experience any side effects.

If your migraines occur during ovulation or menstruation, there are many herbs which can ease the hormonal changes which trigger the migraines. **Blessed thistle** is good for balancing hormones. It also improves the flow of oxygen to the brain and aids in circulation. It is recommended for girls going through puberty as well as women with menstrual difficulties. It's sold singly and in combination formulas.

Squawvine is excellent for menstrual and pre-menstrual difficulties. **Red raspberry** is good for menstrual related problems as is **cramp bark**. **False Unicorn** is good for headaches and other feminine problems. **Uva Ursi** is very healing. **Passion Flower** is also recommended for headaches and PMS.

NURSING

Nursing your baby has many advantages over bottle feeding. Breast milk helps protect babies from infections, allergies, speeds bonding and is easier and better digested than formula.

Breast milk contains colostrum, which contains antibodies to many of the diseases the mother has been immunized against and speeds maturation of the baby's immune system. Breast milk also protects against chest and urinary infections. It is a perfect, complete food for infants.

However wonderful breastfeeding is, there are some occasioanl problems which can occur. Babies eating habits can change, leading to too little milk. Stress and dieting can affect milk production, nipples frequently become sore to the point of being unable to continue breastfeeding. Fortunately, there are things you can do to ensure a successful breastfeeding experience, for both your baby and yourself.

The first problem new mothers face is usually cracked, sore nipples. This usually occurs in the first few weeks and it's important to act quickly to alleviate the problem.

First of all, be sure the baby is postitioned to the breast properly. Make sure you're in a comfortable position when nursing. If the baby's ears move as he feeds, he's latched on properly. If the cheeks move in and out, reposition the baby.

When baby stops active feeding, stop nursing. Be sure the baby eats until satisified, as this will give you a longer break between feedings and give your nipples a rest.

Don't wash your breasts with soap, as it is extremely drying. Just rinse breasts with water when showering. Use breast pads—they absorb excess milk and keep the nipples dry. Alternate breasts at feedings and start on a different side each time. You'll notice the baby sucks hardest when starting to feed; this will lessen the strain on the nipples.

Expose your nipples to air as much as possible. Try **buttermilk** and **comfrey** ointment to keep nipples from becoming cracked and sore. If soreness does occur, try **calendula** or **chickweed** ointment, **almond oil**, **wheatgerm oil** or **rose water** to heal. One drop of rose oil in 2 teaspoonsful almond oil is said to be very effective.

Comfrey ointment is touted as the best tissue healer there is. Also try fresh **mullein leaves** boiled slowly in milk for 10 minutes and cooled. Wrap them in gauze and apply for 10-20 minutes or use mullein ointment. All remedies are best used after feeding.

To increase your milk supply, first of all, relax. It is not uncommon for the milk supply to fluctuate, due to missed feedings, stress, not drinking enough fluids, poor nutrition or baby's changing appetite.

Herbs have been used for centuries to stimulate milk production and enhance the milk supply. Try **anise seed, borage, caraway seeds, centuary, cinnamon, comfrey, dill, false unicorn root, fennel seeds, fenugreeek, goat's rue, holy thistle, garlic, marshmallow, melilot, milk thistle, milkwort, nettles, raspberry leaves, saw palmetto, vervain** and **vitex (chaste tree)**. These can be taken in any form, but teas are preferable as an adequate supply of fluids is crucial to milk production. These herbs are very nutritious and some such as fennel, caraway, cinnamon, aniseed and dill relieve tension.

Don't neglect your diet. You will need at least 500 extra calories a day for milk production. By eating maize, oats, barley, peas, beans, onions and nuts, you will improve the quality of your milk and increase supply.

PREGNANCY

Red raspberry should be started as soon as the pregnancy is known and continued throughout the term. Other herbs that are beneficial during pregnancy include:

Alfalfa: rich in all trace minerals.

Dandelion: a natural diuretic and provides a natural source of iron.

Kelp: natural iodine source, also helps keep weight off the middle and hip area.

Avoid these herbs during pregnancy: Aloe vera, Dong Quai, Pennyroyal and Rue.

To stop the nausea of morning sickness, try red raspberry or peppermint tea. Also try catnip tea and tea with ginger. Small, frequent meals are often easier tolerated.

To avoid miscarriage, try false unicorn and lobelia, taken together.

To rectify toxemia, alfalfa, comfrey, red raspberry, yellow dock and vitamin C are recommended.

During the last six weeks of pregnancy, black cohosh, lobelia, red raspberry, squawvine, hibiscus, peppermint and rosehips all make labor and delivery easier. Blue cohosh will also help labor and strengthen the uterus and female organs.

For labor and delivery, blue cohosh is important. Vitamin E will decrease the need for oxygen during labor. Cornsilk promotes labor if it stops. Red raspberry is essential, coordinates uterine contractions, often shortening labor.

To deal with false labor, catnip tea and blue cohosh should help. Walking is also very helpful.

Postpartum and recovery can be eased considerably with the use of nutmeg to help contract the uterus, cayenne and bayberry slow bleeding. If bleeding is severe, yarrow, mistletoe and cornsilk are used. Shepherd's purse helps blood to clot.

SUMMARY

I've tried many of these supplements and herbs to remedy discomforts and generally improve my overall health and well-being with dramatic success. When looking up an solution to any physical problem, don't get hung up on the diagnosis, so much as the symptoms you are trying to alleviate. True, there are few remedies specifically for endometriosis, for example, but the symptoms of painful menstruation, severe PMS, ovarian pain and water retention were manifestations of the ailment I had to deal with on a daily basis.

The name of the ailment didn't bother me, how I felt did. So I had to find something to make me feel better. I wound up using a combination of red raspberry leaf, squawvine, gotu kola, red clover and cleavers. This combination enabled me to get a handle on fluid retention, regulated my periods and relieved both pain and PMS. I may still technically have endometriosis, but I feel so good, I must admit I don't really care.

April 1994

Dear Reader,

When my mother's father died, years before I was born, he had Alzheimer's Disease. He was a very bright guy. A state senator, a self-made millionaire, owner of farmland and iron mines who predicted the processing of low grade iron ore into taconite 50 years before it happened. But Alzheimer's destroyed his genius.

I have always been concerned about Alzheimer's because of him. The drug companies and the medical community that pushes their products have failed absolutely to treat Alzheimer's. They have had not one success. Not one person helped. Millions spent on drugs with side effects worse than the disease. Billions more spent on drugs to subdue patients who can't be healed.

Maybe there's just too much money in warehousing the violent, destructive, vicious people Alzheimer victims can become. Maybe there's so much money in storage, we can't afford a cure. We have to keep making mushrooms.

I have been studying Alzheimer's for 15 years. Yesterday I bought the best book I have seen on the subject: Reducing the Risk of Alzheimer's by Dr. Michael Weiner.

From what I have read, aluminum is the problem. During World War II, some houses were wired with aluminum because copper was scarce. It didn't work because the aluminum's electrical resistance caused them to melt and short circuit.

Maybe aluminum shorts out your brain's electrical circuitry in the same way. Researchers don't know what causes Alzheimer's, but I'll put my money on aluminum.

Aluminum enters our bodies from drinking water, air pollution, antacids, anti-perspirants, canned food, processed cheese, non-prescription drugs, pots & pans, restaurant food, canned pop and beer—it's everywhere.

A friend of mine theorizes that the magnesium shield protecting our brains from alien minerals becomes depleted, allowing aluminum to enter. He chelates the aluminum with a strain of vitamin C he has developed and suggests magnesium supplements to protect the brain.

It makes sense to me.

A hair analysis will reveal your aluminum level, but any level is too high. The question is: how do we get rid of it?

Dr. Weiner names some foods and vitamins that remove aluminum by chelation. Onions, garlic, chives, red pepper (like cayenne), egg yolks, asparagus, lima beans, pea beans, pintos, kidneys, soybeans and other legumes are natural aluminum chelaters. Don't cook them in an aluminum pot. He also says intravenous chelation with EDTA can be helpful.

Gotu Kola is prescribed to prevent senility and Alzheimer's in India, where they have used it as a brain tonic and anti-aging herb forever. It prevents senility—yet it is one of the highest herbs in aluminum content and also very high in vitamin A, another chelater.

Our bodies don't recognize inorganic vitamins and minerals, so we use only 30 percent of them, throw away 50 percent and store 20 percent—in precarious places, like the brain. I think organic aluminum in the Gotu Kola attaches itself to inorganic aluminum in the brain, so the body recognizes them both and sends them to the dumpster.

I take Cayenne red pepper—a proven aluminum chelater—with Gotu Kola every day. I also drink a lot of Gotu Kola/Chaparral tea. Maybe it will help.

Too bad I never got a chance to tell Grandpa.

Take care of yourself,

P.S. Indian proverb: "A leaf or two a day, keeps old age away."

Help Yourself Improve Your Sex Life

By Kelly Quinn

Everyone has times when sex isn't as much fun as we'd like it to be. Sometimes, stress plays a role, sometimes life just wears you out. Other times, there can be a physical reason for sexual dysfunction or impotence.

No matter what the cause, even if things are fine but you'd like to put a bit more zing in your sex life, there are herbs and supplements reputed to do the trick. You can try them one at a time to see what works for you, or try them in a combination as many synergize together to work even better.

Cloves: increase circulation, promote proper digestion and nutrition. They are a mild sexual stimulant. The seeds are used.

Damiana: has stimulating properties, if you know what I mean. It increases the sperm count in men and strengthens the egg in females. Damiana balances hormones in women and is useful in increasing sexual prowess in both sexes who suffer sexual weakness. It is the most popular and safest of all plants used to restore natural sexual function, relieve female problems, frigidity, the symptoms of menopause and prostate problems. The leaves of the plant are used.

Ginseng: is used for energy, endurance and circulation. It is a cure-all herb. A sexual stimulant, ginseng relieves a host of female problems from menopause to menstrual. It fights depression and restores energy. Siberian ginseng is probably the best to start with as it has fewer potential side-effects. Ginseng can make you feel wired or raise your blood pressure, so start slowly to see how you tolerate it. If you notice nothing negative, gradually increase the dosage. The root is used.

Saw palmetto: has a beneficial effect on all glandular tissues. Useful in treating all diseases of the reproductive glands. Even reputed to increase the size of small breasts. A sexual stimulant.

Schizanda: is a Chinese herb which is supposed to enhance sexual performance in men and is safe for long-term use.

Yohimbe: is classified as *unsafe* by Rodale's Illustrated Encyclopedia of Herbs. The bark is used and it's been sniffed, smoked, brewed up as tea and even rubbed on the body for its alleged aphrodisical properties. While it has been used for centuries as a sex aid, and is still in great demand, it has many negative effects which make it an herb we can not recommend unless it is taken under strict medical supervision.

Yohimbe (or Yohimbine) can cause temporary impotence and lowers the blood pressure. It dilates blood vessels of skin and mucus membranes and increases the reflex excitability of the lower region of the spinal cord. A local anesthetic, it's said to be equal to cocaine in its numbing effects, but longer lasting. Yohimbe is also used as a hallucinogen.

There are many cautions for those taking Yohimbe. Never take it at the same time as foods containing the amino acid tyramine. Liver, cheese, red wine, diet aids and decongestants are in this category. Avoid use if you suffer from hypotension, diabetes, heart, liver or kidney disease, nervous disorders—especially schizophrenia. Anxiety reactions and psychosis have been produced by Yohimbe. Symptoms of overdose include weakness, nervous stimulation, followed by fatigue, paralysis, stomach disorders and ultimately, death.

While we've given more space to the dangers of Yohimbe than the other herbs used to improve sexual function and enjoyment, the continuing popularity of the herb necessitates a detailed warning.

Any or all of the herbs previously mentioned (except Yohimbe!) can be taken separately or in combination form. If you're interested in making your own combination, this one from Today's Herbal Health by Louise Tenney might be a good one to try.

This formula is useful for male hormonal problems like impotence. The main impact of the male hormone testosterone is on the emotions. Shortages of testosterone can lead to irritability, anxiety and lack of sleep and an inability to concentrate.

SEXUAL REJUVENATION COMBINATION

Siberian Ginseng: anti-stress, beneficial to heart and circulation, provides energy, contains testosterone.

Echinacea: blood purifier, enhances immune system, good for prostate enlargement and weakness.

Saw palmetto: hormonal herb for reproductive glands, whole system tonic.

Gotu kola: provides energy, alleviates anxiety, strengthens heart, brain and nerves. Balances hormones.

Damiana: helps balance female hormones, stimulates system, increases sperm count, helps fight impotence.

Sarsasparilla: contains progesterone for glandular balance, stimulates circulation, contains male hormones.

Periwinkle: oxygenates the brain, nourishes and stimulates the system.

Garlic: a natural antibiotic, reduces blood pressure, stimulates cell growth and circulation.

Cayenne: synergizes with herbs to boost their effectiveness, wards off disease, increases blood circulation, energy and endurance.

Chickweed: enhances circulation by dissolving plaque from blood vessels, antiseptic properties, useful in frigidity, hot flashes, menopause, sterility, a sexual stimulant.

Supplements

There are certain supplements you may want to add to your diet, or at least recheck your diet to see if you're getting enough. A shortage of certain vitamins or minerals can lead to sexual dysfunction.

Vitamin A: lessens PMS and irritability.

Vitamin B-complex: with an emphasis on Vitamin B-6, helps in hormonal and sugar balance.

Vitamin C and Bioflavonoids: increases capillary strength, enhances immune system.

Vitamin D: relaxes nerves.

Vitamin E: a male hormone energizer, helps build up sex glands for a youthful hormonal balance.

Vitamin F: alleviates female problems.

Zinc: stimulates prostate.

Seeds, sunflower and pumpkin: stimulates male potency and heals prostate problems.

Bee pollen: is reputed to be an all-around energizer, increasing sex drive and response.

While not technically a supplement, it is believed that **Rose oil** is especially useful in women's problems, alleviating tension and anxiety. Actually, when you think about it, a massage with a sweet-smelling oil would tend to relieve anyone's tension and anxiety.

For the most part, finding a solution to a sexual problem or looking for ways to enhance your sex life requires intuition coupled with common sense. When you hear about some wonder-treatment for sexual dysfunction, take a moment to consider why it might work.

For example, oysters are said to be big-time aphrodisiacs. Ever wonder why? It's because they contain healthy amounts of zinc. As do pumpkin and sunflower seeds, artichokes and asparagus, all reputed to work especially well for male sexual problems.

Many of the herbs listed for their sexual properties contain vitamins and minerals. One thing to remember if you're taking herbs is that they are foods. If you want to be sure your diet contains the proper vitamins and minerals, you'd do well to increase your intake of herbs. When you take vitamins as supplements, absorption is a frequent problem. The vitamins and minerals are not easily recognized or processed by the body and you wind up with expensive urine.

When you get your vitamins in food, the proper combination of necessary vitamins and minerals for rapid absorption are already there. Your body is able to recognize, process and use the nutrients it needs to do what you want it to do, whether it be heal itself, increase your sex drive or just improve upon your sense of general health and well-being.

Just as you need to give your body the proper nutritional support to function properly, you must nurture your spirit as well. If you are stressed out, nervous, and just generally upset, a good sex life can be elusive. Focus on ways to leave the world outside the bedroom door.

Learn ways to de-stress. Exercise, although not listed, is one of the best aphrodisiacs. When you exercise, you relieve stress, become more in tune with your body and generally feel much better about yourself and life in general. Studies have shown time and time again that people who exercise have more sex than those who do not. Just taking a walk and getting some fresh air can make all the difference in the world.

Combine a little exercise with herbs like **gotu kola, gingko biloba** and **cayenne** and you should see a rapid improvement in not only your sex life, but life in general.

$\mathcal{H}$ELP $\mathcal{Y}$OURSELF $\mathcal{C}$HOOSE THE $\mathcal{B}$EST $\mathcal{H}$ERBS FOR $\mathcal{K}$IDS

By Kelly Quinn

*K*ids have many ailments throughout childhood. Parents, deluged with warnings about which medications are the best for children, fear giving them something which won't work, may have negative side effects or could lead to major problems (i.e. Reye's Syndrome). Studies have shown that cold medications don't work very well in children under the age of 12. Other studies link the use of aspirin to Reye's Syndrome, an often fatal disease.

Fortunately, there are herbs which are very effective in treating a host of childhood ailments. For kids that have difficulty in swallowing capsules, herbs can be added to applesauce, pureed fruit and made into teas. Capsules can be taken rectally. Next time you have a sick kid, try some of these remedies:

Colic: try catnip, fennel, peppermint either separately or together as a tea. No sugar as that can exacerbate the problem. If nursing, avoid garlic, onions, beans, broccoli and caffeine.

Constipation: prunes either as juice or the fruit can produce speedy results, as can licorice tea. Be sure to increase the amount of fluid the child is consuming daily. Most constipation is due to insufficient intake of fluids. Try to get the kid to eat more bulky fruits and vegetables, apples and broccoli are particularly good. Avoid laxatives or suppositories as much as possible. Aloe juice can alleviate constipation.

Cradle cap: olive oil, vitamin E or aloe rubbed on the scalp and brushed gently should work.

Diaper rash: responds well to mullein leaf, slippery elm taken internally in juice or applied to the affected area as a paste. Garlic, oil, aloe and vitamin E can be applied externally. Add powdered goldenseal or comfrey to baby powder or cornstarch. Expose the affected area to air as much as possible.

Diarrhea: slippery elm, red raspberry leaf tea, fresh apple juice, banana, white or brown rice, water. Slippery elm can be added to boiled milk.

Dry skin: olive oil works well, as does aloe. Rub into affected area frequently, particularly after bathing to seal in moisture.

Ear infection: garlic oil (break open a capsule of the cheap stuff), mullein oil or lobelia extract may be dropped in the ear. Goldenseal capsule can be inserted in rectum.

Fever: feverfew, white willow bark, red raspberry tea and peppermint tea. Lobelia extract can also help break a fever.

Loss of appetite: chamomile or peppermint tea.

Nausea: aloe juice, chamomile tea, peppermint tea. Ginger settles upset stomachs. Try real gingerale, the flatter the better, preferably at room temperature.

Pinworms: chamomile tea. Try raisins soaked in senna tea for older kids.

Restlessness: hops tea, chamomile tea, valerian. One teaspoon of lobelia extract rubbed on back will soothe. A few drops of lobelia extract on the tongue will quiet baby.

Sore throats: sugary, hard candies should be sucked on to keep flow of saliva going and soothe throats. Sugar speeds healing. For older kids, try a dragon cocktail—cayenne, garlic and tomato juice.

Teething: rub lobelia extract on gums. White oak bark tea, aloe vera gel or peppermint oil can also be rubbed on gums. Try giving baby a popsicle or other frozen treat to gnaw on. Cold will soothe inflamed gums. If the kid doesn't have many teeth, even a cold carrot can provide relief.

All of the above remedies are safe and effective. It's usually best to try to use something natural instead of reaching for the over-the-counter medicine, which often can produce adverse effects. If you call a doctor or nurse for advice, try to ask: is there something I might have around the house that I could try? For constipation, for example, lots of warm water coupled with prunes works better than laxatives because the kid's body is allowed to do its job.

A popular misconception is that a low-grade fever is something that must be stopped. Fever is one of the ways the body uses to kill viruses and infections. While fever is indeed a sign that something is amiss and the child is really sick, it's not a bad idea to let a fever run its course. Even high fevers are rarely harmful. If however, a fever continues to climb and does not respond to herbs, cool baths or wrapping the child in cold towels can break the fever. Be sure to push fluids as the child will become dehydrated quickly, which can be more dangerous than the fever itself. Signs of a high or rising fever include chills, shaking, sweating and a lack of response or interest in the world around him.

Most importantly, trust your instincts. If you feel your child is seriously ill, don't hesitate to seek advice. You can call your doctor, a nurse or the local pharmacist. Keep track of all of the child's symptoms, even those that seem minor. Keep in mind other potentially contributing factors. For example, if the child complains of a stomach ache, but hasn't had a bowel movement for awhile, it's probably constipation. This is particularly common after the temperature rises. Don't expect a kid to drink enough fluids.

If it's been a hot, busy day and the kid complains of a headache, it could be a mild case of heat exhaustion. Push fluids, give the kid some feverfew or white willow bark and insist the child rest in a cool place until she feels better.

My doctor used to call me Dr. Mom. He was making the point that the best way to keep a child healthy is for the parents to take control of the kid's health. Parents know when their kid isn't feeling up to par. If they jump on the first sign of illness, it lessens the duration and severity of the sickness and hastens recovery time.

It's also not a bad idea to pick up some books on children's illnesses. Many times I've found the facts I was looking for by looking up my child's symptoms in such a book. It's also amazing how many illnesses kids get which while they may seem bizarre and serious, simply need to run their course. The knowledge provided in many books can be a great comfort to parents.

> *"Our natures are the physicians of our diseases. This tendency to natural cure should be fostered, with all emphasis on diet and few drugs."*
> —Hippocrates, 460BC

MAKE YOUR KITCHEN YOUR FIRST-AID KIT

By Kelly Quinn

Everyone says you're supposed to have a first-aid kit. But when they tell you what to put in it, it's usually things you'd have to go buy and really, how many people remember to put together a kit full of things they don't normally use, except in emergencies? I know I don't. I have a hard enough time remembering to buy the things I need almost every day without also buying gauze, bandages, etc.

Imagine my delight to discover that without buying anything, I have the makings of a bang-up first-aid kit, right in my kitchen! You do, too! Just make sure you have most of these essentials on hand and you can consider yourself prepared.

Bread: Everyone has bread. You can use it to make a poultice of breadcrumbs which have been put in hot water or milk until they have swollen. Apply as hot as possible. Use the poultice to treat sore muscles, stomach ache, anything you'd use a heat pack for.

Flour or Starch: You probably have flour or cornstarch. Boil some in water and make a poultice for stomachaches, abscesses.

Honey: You can use it to treat a sore throat, put it on an abrasion, or as a laxative for constipation when mixed with warm water.

Lemon: Gargle the juice with warm water for tonsilitis. For wounds and sores, use water flavored with lemon. Lemon is also good for the skin, and eating a lemon is a remedy for a bad cold.

Milk: Soothing to skin, also makes an excellent eyewash. Wash the eyes and then put some drops of warm milk into them.

Mustard: For congestion, make a mustard plaster. Wet a handkerchief with vinegar, fold it and cover it with mustard which you spread with a knife. We're not talking mustard powder here, we mean the mustard you'd put on a hot dog. For fainting or a sick headache, mix some mustard with vinegar and inhale the mixture. Also helps clear the sinuses.

Potato: For burns, grate the pulp of a potato and apply it to the burn. Cover the area with a cloth soaked in oil. Repeat the operation until pain is gone. The potato pulls the heat from the burn, the oil adds moisture.

Salad oil: Make a dressing for a burn or anything you'd want a Band-Aid for by mixing it with flour. For wounds and sores, where you'd want a dressing, wash the wound with wine or vinegar and cover it with a compress impregnated with the oil. Any kind will do, but olive is light and highly recommended.

Thyme: Use about half an ounce of thyme to a quart of water for colds, bronchitis, influenza, stomach problems with fever, even intestinal worms. For sores and gangrene (though I must admit I'd be leery of trying this for gangrene unless there was no way I could get to a doctor), to make antiseptic dressings, use thyme in infusions (boil it and let it steep as it cools) or soaked in wine or vinegar.

Vinegar: Use as a dressing for sores, insect and snake bites (although, once again, it is crucial to get the snake bite victim to the doctor!). For fainting, hold some vinegar under the fainter's nose. Repeat frequently until patient regains and keeps senses. At the same time, dab the temples and neck with vinegar. After spell has passed, pour half a teaspoonful of vinegar into a half pint (one cup) of cold wate and have the patient sip slowly.

Water (*cold*): Soak towels in it and wrap a person with a high fever in them to break the fever and keep it down. For fainting, sprinkle the face with cold water, at the same time rubbing it on the temples. Also apply compresses to the nape of the neck, change frequently. As a diuretic, take cold water with a few drops of lemon juice at bedtime. To control strong emotions and anger, drink a glass of cold water as slowly as possible. To treat loss of appetite, take a glass of cold water with some lemon juice in it half an hour before meals.

Water (*hot*): To cleanse the stomach, take a coffee cupful of hot water, flavored with lemon juice in the morning before breakfast. To aid stomachaches, hot water may be used instead of a poultice. Hot baths aid cramps, sore muscles, induce sleep. To aid constipation, drink as much hot water as possible, approximately 32 ounces.

Water (*warm*): To induce vomiting, take a glass of warm water and cause vomiting by tickling the back of the throat with a finger or even better, the end of a feather.

Wine: Wine is a good dressing for wounds and sores, either by itself or infused with thyme. For stiffness or influenza, lie down and drink a large glass of warm wine, heated until the surface is white, in which some pieces of thyme have been infused. If possible, add some slices of lemon and sweeten with honey. Then cover patient with blankets and keep warm.

Frozen food: If you need an ice pack, for sprains or bruises for example, you 'll find that ice from the freezer is messy, the wrong size to work comfortably and melts quickly. Instead, grab something frozen (vegetables are ideal) and wrap in a thin towel. Apply to infected area until it starts to thaw (you can tell because it becomes pliable) then get something else, refreezing first pack.

Cayenne: Stop bleeding immediately with cayenne. Works internally as well. Stops pain and can stop a heart attack if mixed with a little water and sipped by the patient.

Some of these remedies are a bit unusual, from *The Book of Herbs* by Edmond Bordeaux Sze'kely. He says he used them with great success at a health center in Mexico. Unusual or not, when there is an emergency, being able to take immediate action can mean all the difference in the potential severity of the crisis. Especially if there is no way to seek medical assistance. If the emergency is life-threatening, always seek medical assistance as soon as possible.

In the meantime, post this on the inside of a kitchen cabinet and you'll know you have the information you need to treat emergencies as they arise.

> *"If the doctor heals your wound,*
> *but it breaks out anew because of his*
> *carelessness, neglect or gross want of*
> *skill, he must return the fee you paid.*
> *He must also pay you damages,*
> *if he himself has harmed you.*
> —Ancient Irish Law, compiled by Mary Dowling Daley

HELP YOURSELF AVOID ANTIBIOTIC OVERTREATMENT

By Kelly Quinn

The March 28, 1994 issue of *Newsweek* profiled a problem we've been hearing about for quite some time. It sounds like the plot from a science-fiction movie: bacteria mutate to the point where science has had to come up with stronger and stronger antibiotics to kill them. Finally, the day comes when antibiotics aren't enough, and the bacteria start winning, killing people with what used to be simple infections.

It's not a movie. It's happening right now. Since the discovery of penicillin in 1928, man and microbe have been in a race. But the lead keeps changing. Just five years after penicillin came into wide use, doctors discovered staphylococcus that was invulnerable to the drug. At the time it was a minor problem, scientists invented or discovered new, stronger antibiotics. The drugs pounded the microbes into submission. But the bacteria have always regrouped, and mutants capable of fighting off the latest drugs keep appearing.

Overall, the drugs have retained a slight lead and scourges such as tuberculosis, bacterial pneumonia, septicemia, syphilis, gonorrhea and other bacterial infections appeared vanquished. According to an article on the topic in Newsweek, it looks like medicine declared victory and went home too soon.

Every disease-causing bacterium now has versions that resist at least one of medicine's 100-plus antibiotics. Drug-resistant tuberculosis now accounts for one in seven new cases; 5% of those patients are dying. In 1992, 13,300 hospital patients died of bacterial infections that resisted antibiotics doctors used against them, according to the Centers For Disease Control And Prevention. It wasn't that they were immune to every drug, rather that by the time doctors found an antibiotic that worked, the rampaging bacteria had poisoned the patient's blood, scarred the lungs or crippled some vital organ.

Bacteria develop resistance to antibiotics as a natural part of evolution. When a colony of bacteria is hit with penicillin, for example, most die. But a few microbes, just by chance, harbor mutant genes which make them immune to the drug. The mutants then pass on their resistance genes to their progeny. One bacterium can leave 16,777,220 offspring within just 24 hours. More insidious, the mutants even share the resistance gene with unrelated microbes. So while antibiotics didn't create resistance genes, the drugs fast-forwarded their spread.

Even more frightening is that the germs can become resistant to antibiotics they've never been exposed to. In women receiving tetracycline for a urinary tract infection, E. coli developed resistance not only to tetracycline, but to other antibiotics too.

Scary, isn't it? Of course, this is all in addition to the problems which are common side-effects of antibiotic use. Allergic reactions such as rashes, nausea and headache are relatively common. Any female who takes antibiotics at some point will discover the discomfort of yeast infections as antibiotics kill off friendly bacteria as well as unfriendly, resulting in an overgrowth of yeast. Fungal infections and thrush are also common side-effects of antibiotic use.

Scientists have been trying to come up with a strategy to break the bacterial stronghold. Researchers are looking at drugs which increase the acidity in the intestine, figuring they can be killed off by creating a more hostile environment. Another idea is designing vaccines to work against bacteria — there already is a vaccine against pneumococus. But research on vaccines against strep and staph is nearly nonexistent. Vaccines aren't big revenue generators, so research money goes elsewhere, to something that has a bigger pay back.

So, what's a person to do? Before the advent of the "Superbugs," if you had to break down and take antibiotics, you could at least feel pretty confident that they'd cure whatever the infection was. These days, you can't always be sure of that. Fortunately, there are indeed herbs which contain natural antibiotics. Herbs can be just as efficacious as antibiotics, but with fewer side-effects if taken properly.

According to the book *Fighting Infections With Herbs* by Linda

Rector-Page N.D., Ph.D, there are four major types of infections:

Bacterial: usually an infection by a pathenogenic micro-organism, but may also be an opportunistic infection. Examples of bacterial infections include upper respiratory infections, bacterial cystitis, bacterial sinusitis, abscesses and acne.

Herbs recommended for bacterial infections include: Echinacea, Goldenseal, Myrrh, Garlic, Pau de Arco, Chaparral, Elecampane and Black Walnut Hulls.

Viral: are infections by a simple, living organism with a rapid reproductive mechanism and the ability to move and mutate in order to avoid being overcome by the body's defense system. Viral infections are virulent, deep reaching and tenacious. Antibiotics are ineffective against viruses, but herbs bring good results.

Examples of viral infections include: genital warts, Epstein Barr Virus (chronic fatigue syndrome), AIDS, Herpes, Hepatitis and Pneumonia.

Anti-viral herbs include St. John's Wort, Astragalus, Reishi Mushrooms, Chaparral, Echinacea, Garlic, Myrrh, Honeysuckle and Comfrey Root.

Fungal Infections: are infections by a fungus microbe. Characterized by moist, weepy, red patches on the body. Stimulating and rebuilding the immune response is the key to control. Examples of fungal infections include: Athletes Foot, Vaginitis, Ringworm, Thrush and Candidiasis.

Anti fungal herbs include **Myrrh, Black Walnut Hulls, Tea Tree Oil**, Chaparral, Barberry, Goldenseal, Garlic and Wormwood.

Parasitic Infections: are and infection by a parasite resulting in weakening of the entire body system. Examples of parasitical infections include: Amoebic Dysentery, Malaria, Sleeping Sickness, Giadia, Trichomonas, Hookworms, Roundworms, Whipworms and Tapeworms.

Anti-parasite herbs include Myrrh, Black Walnut Hulls, Chaparral, Garlic, Barberry, Wormwood, Tansy, Pau de Arco, Mullein, Echinacea, Chamomile and Valerian.

Herbal Formulas

Herbs are at their best in formulas. The herbs in a well-crafted compound work together as a whole, synergistically, to concentrate on the different aspects of a problem. Try some of the following formulas next time you're troubled by an infection:

Staph Infection is usually virulent and often food-borne. You can suspect food poisoning, staph infection if you have nausea, vomiting, stomach cramps and diarrhea within two to six hours after eating. Other common staph infections cause skin sores such as boils and abscesses. Herbal therapy centers on destroying and flushing the active microbe from the body. Use all during healing: **Garlic** capsules, two, three times daily. **Echinacea/Goldenseal/Myrrh** extract, 15 drops two times a day. **Propolis** twice a day to support immune system response.

A **Sore Throat, Streptococcal Infection** can be managed symptomatically. Herbal formulas work quickly if begun at the onset of symptoms. Lack of toxicity makes them an easy first-line defense. In most cases, you don't even need to differentiate between a bacterial and viral condition because herbs with multi anti-infective activity can be used. An effective antibiotic formula for sore or strep throat might look like this: **Echinacea Angustifolia** and **Purpurea, Goldenseal Root, Myrrh, Propolis**. A **green tea** cleansing drink is another option. It contains effective tannins which are astringent and anti-bacterial, and help eliminate mucus and reduce infection. An immune-activating tea should be taken each morning and could look like this: **Bancha Green Tea Leaves, Gotu Kola, Burdock Root, Fo-Ti-Tieng, Kukicha Twig, Hawthorn Berry, Orange Peel, Cinnamon.**

A **Gardnerella Vaginal Infection** is a bacterial microbe that thrives when vaginal pH is disturbed. It is usually transmitted through sexual contact. Gardnerella is characterized by an especially foul, fishy odor, creamy white discharge and moderate itchiness. Effective natural therapies for gardnerella would include:
• Two glasses of sugar-free cranberry juice daily
• Insert a **Tea Tree Oil** vaginal suppository nightly for two weeks or douche with 1/2 teaspoonful Tea Tree Oil in one quart water.
• Avoid **caffeine** and **refined sugars** until body balance is restored.
• **Vitamin B complex**, 100 mg. and **Vitamin C**, up to 5000 mg. daily.
• Add the following herbal antibiotic formula: **Goldenseal Root, Myrrh, Pau d'Arco, Echinacea Angustifolia, Vegetable Acidophilus.**

Bacterial Cystitis Infections are common in women because of the proximity of the bladder and the urethra to the vagina. Most UTIs also involve a mild to serious kidney infection, making the problem progressively worse. Prompt attention to the first signs of a UTI are necessary to avoid rapid deterioration. Herbal therapies can help in all stages with many types of bladder infections. Herbal therapy for a UTI is four-fold: 1) demulcent herbs to soothe the tissues, 2) herbs to reduce inflammation, 3) plants with antibiotic activity, 4) herbs to flush toxins from the body.

An effective capsule with these properties would look like this: Juniper Berry, Parsley Root, Goldenseal Root, Uva Ursi, Marshmallow Root, Dandelion Leaf, Stone Root, Mullein, Ginger Root, Hydrangea, Vitamin B6, Lobelia.

Chronic Fatigue Syndrome (CFS) may result from immune suppression setting the stage for **Epstein-Barr Virus (EBV)**. In fact CFS itself acts like a recurring systemic viral infection and EBV may be only one of several viruses involved. CFS does not respond to conventional medical treatment and many drugs on the market actually hinder immune response and recovery. Liver health is the key to overcoming CFS. An herbal formula should be included for the first three months. Try: **Beet Root, Milk Thistle Seed, Oregon Grape, Dandelion Root, Wild Yam, Yellow Dock, Licorice, Ginkgo Biloba, Barberry, Gotu Kola, Ginger, Wild Cherry Bark.** Some herbs can attack the virus directly. An extract of **Lomatium** and **St. John's Wort** is imperative as part of the herbal program.

Chronic Hepatitis is a good example of the rapidity and severity with which viruses mutate, replicate, grow and are passed in society. Natural therapy works at the cause of the infection, rather than the individual virus. The following simplified program offers a good diet and natural therapy start to build on. A cleansing, balancing diet lays the foundation for healing elements to work. Avoid meat protein, refined, fried and fatty foods, sugars, alcohol and caffeine. Herbal therapy is focused on healing and rebuilding the liver. For the first two weeks to one month, both capsules and a tea should be taken. The capsule should include as many of the following herbs as possible: **Beet Root, Milk Thistle Seed, Oregon Grape, Dandelion Root, Wild Yam, Yellow Dock, Licorice, Ginkgo Biloba, Barberry Bark, Gotu Kola, Ginger, Wild Cherry Bark.** The tea should be taken twice daily and might look like this: **Dandelion, Watercress, Yellow Dock, Pau d'Arco, Hyssop, Parsley Leaf, Oregon Grape, Red Sage, Licorice, Milk Thistle, Hibiscus.**

For the second month of healing, reduce the dosage of the preceding in half and add a blood-building compound. It should contain some of these herbs: **Beet Root, Alfalfa, Dandelion, Yellow Dock, Bilberry, Parsley Root, Nettles, Burdock, Dulse, Siberian Ginseng, Capsicum (Red Pepper).**

An **Herbal Anti-Fungal** program for chronic Athletes Foot or Nail Fungus would include these choices taken twice daily in capsule form: Burdock, Bayberry, Dandelion, Black Walnut Hulls, Gentian, Uva Ursi, Parsley Root, Juniper Berry, Squawvine. You can also apply Tea Tree Oil on the affected areas several times daily. Most people notice improvement within one week and healing within three to six weeks.

Herbal Parasiticides are a good choice for chronic, mild parasite infestation. **Giardia** is the most prevalent parasite in the U.S. and the number one cause of the water-borne disease. Herbs treat underlying deficiencies and rebuild strength. However, they are very slow working in cases of heavy parasite infection. A better protocol in serious cases is to use herbs for cleansing and rebuilding the tissues after a short course of antibiotic drugs. A good herbal program might include **Black Walnut Hulls** extract, four times daily with **Barberry Tea** as an anti-infective. Add two to four **Garlic** capsules daily and a compound like this: **Black Walnut Hulls, Garlic, Pumpkin, Butternut Bark, Cascara Sagrada, Mugwort, False Unicorn, Gentian Root, Slippery Elm, Wormwood, Fennel.**

Sexually Transmitted Diseases

Chlamydia has reached epidemic proportion in the U.S. In addition to being a sexually transmitted disease, this bacteria-like parasite is the leading cause of blindness in humans. It is the most harmful of all STD's in terms of infertility for both men and women. Blood cleansing herbs have been effective against chlamydia infection. Treatment should be started as soon as infection is known and should continue for one to three months. A strong blood cleansing compound might look like this: **Red Clover, Licorice, Burdock, Pau d'Arco, Echinacea Purpurea, Ascorbate Vitamin C, Garlic, Kelp, Alfalfa, Dandelion Root, Poria Mushroom, American Ginseng, Sarsaparilla Root, Astragalus Bark, Yellow Dock, Butternut Bark, Prickly Ash, Buckthorn Bark, Milk Thistle Seed, Goldenseal.** Diluted Goldenseal tea may be used as an effective eyewash to kill the chlamydia parasite. The same tea may be used on infected genitals.

Herpes Simplex Virus 2 is the most widespread of all STDs, affecting between 50 and 100 million Americans. It is a life-long infection which alternates between virulent and quiescent stages. Symptoms include headache, stiff neck, fever, pain, swelling and itching in the genital area, genital blisters that swell and become festering ulcers and shooting pains through the thighs and legs. An outbreak lasts from one to two weeks. Herbal treatment has had marked success in treating herpes. Effective herbs to reduce frequency of outbreaks and reduce pain of symptoms might include these:

To neutralize toxins, strengthen liver function and cleanse the blood try Astragalus, L-lysine, Gentian Root, Bupleurum, Poria Mushroom, Yellow Dock, Echinacea Angustifolia, Red Sage, Myrrh, Wild Yam, Sarsaparilla, Oregon Grape, Marshmallow Root, Vitamin E. Use over a three to six month period for best results.

To reduce inflammation and swelling, try: White Willow, Echinacea Purpurea and Angustifolia, St. John's Wort, Gotu Kola, Red Clover, Devil's Claw, Burdock Root, Dandelion, Chamomile, Yucca, White Pine Bark, Alfalfa, Ginger Root, Bromelain 60 mg.

Genital Warts are caused by the human papilloma virus and are the most contagious STD. Natural therapy for genital warts takes about 6 months. It is especially successful for women with precancerous conditions of the cervix and focuses on a three pronged attack: topical applications, herbal anti-virals and immune system support.

Vaginal packs may be applied via herbal suppository or tampon placed against the cervix and include the following:

A solution of **chlorella, spirulina** or **barley grass**.

An internal poultice pack to draw out infective wastes that might look like this: **Cranesbill, Goldenseal, Raspberry Leaf, White Oak Bark, Echinacea Root, Myrrh Gum**. For best results, apply at night upon retiring and rinse each morning with a douche of **Yellow Dock** or **White Oak Bark Tea**. Wear a sanitary napkin to catch drainage as infective wastes are released. Abstain from sexual intercourse during pack treatment.

Effective topical applications for men include the following: **Aloe Vera Gel** (and two glasses of **Aloe Vera Juice** daily) and **Oxygel** applied twice daily.

An effective immune support program for both men and women might include two herbal compounds, an extract to overcome replication of the virus: **Lomatium Dissectum, St. John's Wort, Bupleurum**, or **Cinnamon**; and a heating formula to slightly raise body temperature during acute stages: **Bayberry, Rose Hips, Vitamin C, White Pine Bark, White Willow Bark, Ginger Root, Cloves** and **Capsicum (Cayenne)**. The two compounds should be taken together, one week on and one week off until improvement is felt.

Trichomonas is a common, sexually transmitted parasitic infection that affects both men and women. It produces burning, itching and genital discharge. Unfortunately, the standard medical treatment, metronidazole, can cause cancer and birth defects. Natural therapies are effective and free of side-effects. Many people who have trichomonas have low Zinc levels. To increase the amount of Zinc naturally, try an herbal formula such as this: **Echinacea Angustifolia, Spirulina, Gotu Kola, Yellow Dock, Peppermint, Alfalfa, Barley Grass, Bilberry**. Since this is a bacteria-like organism, herbal antibiotic treatment can be helpful. Two separate formulas should be used alternately to produce the strength and broad-spectrum activity needed.

1. Goldenseal, Myrrh Gum, Pau d'Arco, Echinacea Angustifolia, Vegetable Acidophilus.
2. Burdock Root, Bayberry, Dandelion, Black Walnut Hulls, Gentian, Uva Ursi, Parsley Root, Juniper Berry, Squawvine.

Summary

There are a few pointers for taking herbal antibiotic and antiparasitic treatments. Also from Linda Rector-Page's book *Fighting Infections With Herbs/Sexually Transmitted Infections,* are these hints:

• Take the formula for your condition at the right time—not all the time—for best results.
• Rotating and alternating herbal combinations according to your health goals will allow the body to remain most responsive to their effects.
• Take herbs in descending strength, and rest on the seventh day each week.
• Start with greater amounts at the beginning of your program. As your health returns, fewer and fewer of the large initial doses should be taken.
• Most people realize an herbal treatment has done its job when they forget to take it.
• Give herbs time to work.

Antibiotics still have a place in healing. If the illness is severe, or you find yourself growing concerned, never hesitate to seek professional advice. There are times when an antibiotic might work faster and therefore more effectively on an illness. In the case of some illnesses, strep for example, it is wise to work hand-in-hand with your doctor. Strep can affect the heart and lead to rheumatic fever. If the patient appears to be getting worse, consult a doctor. Doctors have an important role in healing. The wise patient explores all available avenues, choosing the easiest and least toxic paths to wellness.

ℋERBS TO ℐILENCE ℐINNITUS

By Dick Quinn

Tinnitus, ringing in the ears, is a problem that plagues many, bringing insomnia, stress, confusion, and sometimes headaches. It's often caused by high blood pressure, hypoglycemia (low blood sugar), nutritional deficiencies, and chemical imbalance.

Major herbs for treatment: black cohosh, garlic, goldenseal (lowers blood sugar), gotu kola, hawthorn, horsetail, skullcap, valerian (safely relaxing), and wood betony. From Health Handbook by Louise Tenney.

Black cohosh is recommended by Daniel B. Mowrey in *Scientific Validation of Herbal Medicine,* but other herbalists say it can cause slowed or irregular heartbeat. Since the most important ingredients in black cohosh are water soluble resins, it is very effective as a tea. One cup a day would seem to be a safe dose, unless you have low blood pressure, slow pulse, arrhythmia, or irregular heartbeat. The herb's ancillary benefits make it ideal for women over 40.

Mistletoe tea is effective against tinnitus. Take 1 or 2 cups daily. *From Family Herbal* by Peter and Barbara Theiss.

Feverfew combats tinnitus and migraine headaches. It is known to be heart-safe. Take it as a tea (2 cups daily), or in capsules (2-4 daily).

Ginkgo biloba is also recommended by herbalists who suggest two or more capsules daily of guaranteed potency concentrate.

> *"Half the modern drugs could well be thrown out the window, except that the birds might eat them."*
> —Martin H. Fischer, 1879-1962

$\mathcal{H}$ERBS TO $\mathcal{T}$REAT $\mathcal{M}$ULTIPLE $\mathcal{S}$CLEROSIS

By Dick Quinn

Multiple sclerosis is a degenerative disorder requiring a diet free of sugar, coffee, alcohol, chocolate, caffeine, and refined foods. Drug therapies have been largely unsuccessful and patients have experimented with bee venom and other alternatives with limited success. Vitamins C, E, and F are recommended by nutritionists, as are inositol, calcium, iron, magnesium, manganese, selenium, and zinc. Some herbs have also proven effective.

Skullcap, the non-toxic herb that's very high in copper, builds the central nervous system. Combine it with valerian, the high-calcium herb, and mineral-rich kelp for nutritional balance and stress protection. Ashwagandha, the ayurvedic herb called "Indian Ginseng," provides healing energy. Many herbalists also recommend passion flower, the Parkinson's Disease herb, and lobelia, the herbal relaxant.

Marijuana relieved fatigue, stopped tremors and spasms, and seemed to deter attacks in studies of MS patients by M. Dunn and R. Davis, reported in *Parapalegia* (#12, 1974, pg. 175) and by Denis J. Petro for *Psychosomatics,* (#21, 1980, pages. 81, 85). It also has proven effective in deterring epileptic attacks.

Evening primrose oil is said to rebuild nerve sheaths damaged by MS. Lecithin is also said to aid in this process.

> "Better to hunt in the fields for
> Health unbought, than fee the doctor
> for a nauseous draught.
> —John Dryden, 1631-1700, FABLES ANCIENT AND MODERN

How I Finally Quit Smoking

By Dick Quinn

The first cigarettes I ever had was a pack of Chesterfields a friend of mine stole. I was 6. After that, I rolled cigarettes, bummed cigarettes and occasionally bought cigarettes. I even smoked Red Dot cigars for a while. They were "wine dipped" and cost only a nickel—what a deal.

For years I smoked Pall Malls, then Benson & Hedges. Finally, when I was 30, I switched to hand rolled cigarettes made from Bugler tobacco, thinking it would cut down my nicotine consumption, which it did. When I was 35, I decided to quit. It was a five year struggle and I probably would never have succeeded had I not discovered a non-tobacco cigarette called Free, made from coconut husks. Free cigarettes satisfied my urge to smoke and, since they came in a real package, I wasn't kicked out of bars and restaurants for "smoking dope," as happened when I smoked herbal cigarettes. Free cigarettes smoked so well, in fact, the tobacco companies put them out of business.

That was in 1976, the year I finally quit. What a struggle. In October 1978, I began taking Cayenne red pepper, which made me allergic to tobacco, so I can never go back. That part is terrific. I can't be around tobacco without becoming instantly sick. It's a wonderful allergy; everybody should have it.

But it's fun to smoke, so I still experiment with herbal cigarettes occasionally. Some are pretty good and some are terrible. I don't think inhaling smoke is good for anybody, but I also realize non-tobacco cigarettes helped me kick a tobacco addiction that was killing me.

Some herbs can help you stop smoking. As I mentioned, I became allergic to tobacco after I began taking Cayenne. According to recent research on plant chemicals, Cayenne also contains a substance which can prevent carcinogens in cigarette smoke from uniting with DNA to cause lung cancer. Cayenne also boosts your metabolism, which counters the tendency to gain weight when you quit smoking.

Hops, Slippery Elm, Valerian and Skullcap kill the desire for tobacco when taken together. Slippery Elm lozenges reportedly stop the craving for tobacco, as do carrots—eat at least two or three daily. Studies at a Scottish hospital showed that oat plant extract helped smokers cut down and quit much more successfully than the placebo. Put about 10 drops under your tongue three to four times daily.

Tobacco is an herb and all herbs have buffering or counter herbs. The buffer for tobacco is Lobelia.

The herb Lobelia contains a substance called lobeline, which the body mistakes for nicotine, alleviating the craving. It was in all the non-prescription stop-smoking formulas until the FDA restricted its sale to pave the way for the nicotine patch. The flowers can be smoked, taken as a whole herb in capsules or as a tincture (several drops under the tongue whenever needed).Lobelia also relaxes the bronchial area to relieve asthma, but it can cause nausea in large doses. Catnip is a mood elevating herb that calms smokers' nerves. In capsules, tea or smoke it.

Perhaps the true super weapon against tobacco is sunflower seeds. According to John Heinerman's *Encyclopedia of Fruits, Vegetables and Herbs,* tobacco smoke triggers the release of stored glycogen sugar from your liver that works quickly to perk up your brain pleasurably. It's the tobacco rush that makes us want to smoke. Raw, shelled sunflower seeds trigger the same sugar release, answering the craving.

Tobacco has a sedating or calming effect; so do sunflower seeds, which are high in the B vitamins that nourish the nervous system. Sunflower seeds also boost the output of adrenal gland hormones, as tobacco does, to control allergies and respiratory problems that often emerge when one quits smoking.

Some herbs are especially effective when chewed, perhaps because of their effect on blood sugar and the liver.

Chinese Licorice Root can be chewed. It's very, very sweet, a stimulant that lowers blood sugar, stimulates estrogen and acts on the liver. Licorice is not used in licorice candy, which is made with anise also an herb. Colombo root, Gentian root, Calamus root and Chamomile flowers are all said to kill the urge when chewed.

Fresh fruit (especially apples) and honey are said to stop craving.

Fruit at the end of the meal curbs desire for an after dinner smoke. To speed the nicotine from the blood stream, drink lots of water and take Burdock Root in capsules or tea (it's too bitter to chew).

In *Back to Eden,* Jethro Kloss says Magnolia, Peppermint, Vervain, Motherwort, Quassia chips, Blue and Black Cohosh and Sweet Flag are all herbs that control the desire for nicotine. You can take them as tea or in capsules. Not all are safe during pregnancy.

Burdock root cleans the blood of tobacco's toxins when taken as tea or in capsules. Chew Sassafras root or make Sassafras tea to kill the urge.

Weight gain is a major problem for many who quit smoking. Cayenne helps by boosting the metabolism, much as tobacco does. Guar gum is a proven dieting herb that also lowers cholesterol; two 4 to 6 capsules daily. The Ayurvedic herb Guggalo lowers cholesterol and helps rid the body of fat. If sugar is your downfall, Gymnama Sylvestre (also called Gurmar) is an Ayurvedic herb from India that causes the body to excrete up to 60% of the sugar consumed. The Gurmar molecule unites with the sugar molecule, so neither can pass through the walls of the intestine to be absorbed.

I went on a very low carbohydrate diet when I finally quit smoking, and actually lost 20 pounds. Tobacco is an herb, but there are many other non-addictive herbs that can be smoked in pipes and rolled into cigarettes. Here are some ideas from *Mastering Herbalism* by Paul Huson, *Herbs for Healthful Living* by Richard Lucas, *The Healing Power of Herbs* by May Bethel, personal experience and other sources.

According to the *Historical Dictionary* of 1813, Native Americans from the Western states mixed Sumach Berries and leaves equally to make a smoking mixture called Kinikah, which killed the desire for tobacco. Corn Silk is a valuable medicinal herb used for kidney, bladder and prostate disorders, that's also found in some herbal smoke mixtures.

Colombo Root, which stops craving, smokes well as does Comfrey Root, which is said to have a healing effect on the lungs. Some people mix herbs with pipe tobacco to gradually reduce nicotine intake. Coltsfoot, Rosemary, Eyebright, Thyme and Chamomile all smoke well. I have found that Passion Flower makes a very mild, pleasant smoke. Gentian and Sweet Clover also smoke well. Native Americans smoked Corn Silk, Sassafras and Mullein with and without tobacco.

According to Leonard Herter's *Bull Cookbook,* stop the tobacco craving by going through the day with an un-lit cigarette in your mouth.

The leaves of Bearberry (or Uva Ursi), Buckbean, Chervil, Dittany, Eyebright, Life Everlasting, Marjoram, Raspberry, Sage and Wood Betony are all smoked. Lavender flowers and Rose petals and Chamomile flowers can be added for a nice aroma.

Not all herbs are safe to smoke, so be cautious in your experimentation. But it is hard to find anything more poisonous than tobacco.

Good luck!

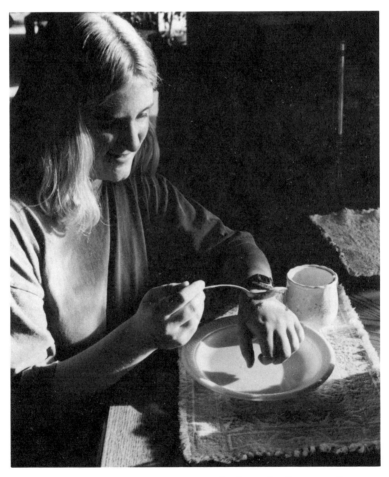

Heather treats a minor cut with sugar for faster healing. It's also very effective for treating burns.

HELP YOURSELF CHOOSE THE RIGHT FORMULA

By Kelly Quinn

*I*magine yourself looking through the displays at a health store. Rows and rows of different products confront you. You thought you knew what you wanted, but now you're not so sure. The labels of most herbal preparations have little connection with the intended purpose of the formula. Yes, you can buy the herbs separately and combine them as needed, but if you take a lot of herbs, that can mean a lot of capsules to swallow.

So you'd like a combination formula, something where the herbs are already mixed together in the right amounts. Sounds good doesn't it? Until you try to find one.

For example, what in the world is BF & C Formula? How about AKN Formula? These are actual products by Nature's Way. We're going to make it easier for you to get the products you need by going through different products, their names, and their uses. Hopefully, next time you go into a health store, you'll know exactly what you want and be able to ask for the product by name.

If you're lucky, the product will still exist. Case in point: I purchased a Nature's Way formula called Rheum-Aid. When I went to get more, I found the product no longer existed. Now, it's called Yucca-AR. Same stuff, same use, different name. But, since I know what's in the formula, I was able to find a similar product while I tracked down the original. You'll notice frequent name changes as well.

First, let's tackle the **Nature's Way** product line, predominant in most stores, even in some drugstores. If you're looking for single herbs, they have a picture of the herb and list it by name. Easy enough, but if you're looking for a combination, you'll need help.

ADR-NL *(previously known as AdrenAid Formula)*: contains Mullein Leaves, Licorice Root, Gotu Kola, Cayenne, Ginger Root, Siberian Ginseng and Hawthorn Berries.

What's it used for? "A nutritional supplement to ensure a healthy glandular system," according to product literature. Primarily targeted to those with an active lifestyle.

Comments: Licorice Root, Gotu Kola, Cayenne, Ginger and Siberian Ginseng are all stimulants. If you take this, you can expect to feel more energetic, rested. You may also notice an increase in blood pressure due to the Licorice Root.

AKN Formula: contains Dandelion Root, Sarsaparilla Root, Burdock Root, Licorice Root, Echinacea, Yellow Dock, Norwegian Kelp, Cayenne and until recently, Chaparral.

What's it used for? "A supplement to promote healthy skin."

Comments: I would never have guessed this product to be for the skin, although the skin would indeed benefit from the many blood detoxifiers in the product. In fact, every herb except Echinacea is a detoxifier. I would be inclined to take this if I was suffering from an illness and wanted to help my body remove toxins. I'd also take it for water retention. The product would most likely give added energy, but I'd be hesitant to take it long-term, because of the possible increase in blood pressure from the Licorice. Also, it's not a good idea to take Echinacea on a regular basis. A natural antibiotic, Echinacea is better taken for its healing powers. Expect to go to the bathroom a lot when on this combination.

A-P Formula: contains Wild Lettuce, Valerian Root, Cayenne.

What's it used for? A supplement to alleviate headaches, muscle aches, tension.

Comments: Valerian is a key player here. It relaxes tense muscles, reduces the effects of stress. Cayenne provides energy and improves circulation. Personally, I'd be more inclined to take a White Willow Bark combination for pain and simple Valerian for stress and relaxing tense muscles.

APH Formula: contains Damiana Leaves, Siberian Ginseng, Echinacea, Fo-Ti, Gotu Kola, Sarsaparilla and Saw Palmetto.

What's it used for? "A dietary supplement" which helps the body "overcome fatigue."

Comments: Not only should this formulation bring added energy, but it could enhance your sex drive. Damiana, Saw Palmetto, Siberian Ginseng, Sarsaparilla and Fo-Ti are all used for their aphrodisiacal properties. The addition of Echinacea is the only herb I'd have a problem with, because it's not always wise to take it for extended periods. If you were to take this combination only occasionally rather than on a regular basis, that would be fine. But chances are, the combination of the other herbs would make this a supplement you'd want to take on a daily basis. If so, you'd be wise to look for a similar supplement without Echinacea.

B/P Formula: contains Cayenne, Parsley, Ginger, Goldenseal, Garlic and Siberian Ginseng.

What's it used for? A nutritional supplement to promote improved circulation. I imagine "B/P" stands for "Blood Pressure."

Comments: Regular use of Goldenseal is not recommended. The other herbs in the formula are good for circulation and synergize extremely well together.

Bee Pollen With Ginseng: contains Bee Pollen with Wild Siberian Ginseng.

What's it used for? The product is promoted as a supplement among athletes and others seeking to maximize their performance.

Comments: You should feel more energy and improved stamina due mostly to the Ginseng. Siberian Ginseng is popular because although it provides most of the benefits of Chinese and Korean Ginseng, it has few of the side-effects. If you take too much of this product, you may feel wired. Cut back if this happens. Bee Pollen has gotten rave reviews as a supplement, even attributing its use to alleviating allergies and improving your sex life. I've taken Bee Pollen and didn't notice any benefits or negative results.

ENER-CHI *(previously known as EnerGizer Formula):* contains: Vitamin E, Korean White Ginseng Root, Bee Pollen, Lecithin and Wheat Germ Oil.

What's it used for? Promoted as a "pick-me-up" to restore energy or relieve simple fatigue.

Comments: The really important ingredient in this formula is the Korean White Ginseng Root. You probably won't notice any difference in how you feel with the other ingredients. Bee Pollen may synergize with the Ginseng to provide some additional energy. None of the ingredients are harmful, Vitamin E, Lecithin and Wheat Germ Oil are nice but nothing spectacular in the amounts they'd be included in the formula. If you are interested in supplementing your diet with Lecithin, Vitamin E or Wheat Germ Oil, you'd be better off buying and taking them separately. Not necessarily a bad formula, just not a particularly beneficial one.

Fenu-Thyme Formula: contains Fenugreek seed and Thyme.
What's it used for? A dietary supplement to assist the body in overcoming minor cold and flu symptoms such as congestion, stuffiness and mucus build-up.
Comments: Both Fenugreek and Thyme are used for colds. Could be helpful, but you may need to increase the dosage from the suggested dose to get results.

Garlic-Parsley Formula: contains Garlic and Parsley.
What's it used for? "A mild herbal diuretic that provides the benefits of Garlic plus Parsley."
Comments: Parsley is the natural deodorizer for Garlic breath. I wouldn't use this as a diuretic, but rather for the many health benefits of Garlic. There are many other much more effective diuretic formulas available.

H Formula: contains Hawthorn Berries, Cayenne, Vitamin E and Lecithin.
What's it used for? A nutritional supplement designed to help provide certain nutrients known to be present in healthy heart and circulation. (*Editor's note:* "Not intended to treat symptoms of heart disease or circulatory problems, or to replace proper medical care."
Comments: The disclaimer says it all. The product is used to prevent and repair damage from circulatory diseases and heart attacks. Hawthorn is the #1 heart strengthening herb, Cayenne flushes arteries and improves circulation, Lecithin helps manage cholesterol and studies have shown Vitamin E helps prevent heart disease. If you know the clues, you can find some interesting products. Basically, if a formula works too well, you'll find they have to be very careful about FDA regulations, or it could be taken off the market. This is a formula everyone should take, every day.

HAS Formula: contains extract of Pseudoephedrine 30 mg., Brigham Tea, Marshmallow Root, Burdock Root, Parsley, Cayenne, Goldenseal and Lobelia. (This product used to contain Chaparral, but alas, no longer.)

What's it used for? Use to open bronchial tubes and ease breathing for temporary relief of bronchial asthma and related symptoms of hay fever and allergies.

Comments: I would not buy this product. I could go to a drug-store and get some generic Sudafed and get the same results. They throw all sorts of wonderful detoxifying and healing herbs in to compensate for the nasty side-effects of a chemical additive. True, Pseudoephedrine does come from the herb Ephedra, also known as Ma Huang, but it can raise blood pressure, increase heart rate and produce anxiety and nervousness. It has stimulant properties, which makes it work against the relaxant Lobelia, or the natural energy produced by Cayenne.

Herbal Influence Formula: contains Bayberry Root, Ginger Root, Garlic, Cayenne and White Pine Bark.

What's it used for? This combination contains herbs used "primarily during the winter months." At least, that's what the product information says about it. Why we'd want to take it in the winter is beyond me. Could be some sort of circulatory and tonic formula, as Garlic, Cayenne and Ginger are heart herbs. White Pine Bark would probably be a system toner of some sort, although it is an obscure herb, not found in many herb books.

Comments: This would be a good herb to fight and prevent heart disease and circulatory problems. You'd also feel more energy due to the Cayenne, Ginger and Garlic.

H-Up Formula: contains Siberian Ginseng Root, Gotu Kola, Bee Pollen, Suma, Hawthorn Berries and Cayenne.

What's it used for? These ingredients support an active lifestyle. Meaning: these caps will give you energy. All the herbs are energy and strength herbs, and work synergistically together.

Comments: This would be an extremely valuable formula for almost anyone. It would give natural, healthy energy and be a good formula to help avoid heart disease, ulcers, impotence and other circulatory ills.

Silent Night Formula: contains Hops, Valerian and Skullcap.

What's it used for? "An herbal supplement for use as a natural nighttime supplement."

Comments: Use this one if you haven't been sleeping very well. Personally, I think the name would be more appropriate for a cough preparation, but this is a good product.

Yellow Dock Combination: contains White Oak Bark, Yellow Dock, Mullein, Black Walnut Hulls, Marshmallow Root and Calendula Flowers.

What's it used for? "A supplement designed to promote general good health," reads the literature, telling us absolutely nothing. I have this product for detoxification purposes. Yellow Dock is a fabulous blood detoxifier, but it can interfere with iron absorption, so you wouldn't want to take this on a daily basis. Mullein, Marshmallow Root and Calendula Flowers are all soothing, healing herbs. White Oak Bark is an all-body toner, anti-inflammatory herb.

Comments: If you've had the flu, for example, you might be inclined to take this product to help your body eliminate toxins and soothe and cleanse your system. You should take a break between bottles. I'd recommend two capsules, three times a day.

Yucca A-R *(formerly Rheum-Aid Formula):* contains Yucca, Wild Yam, Hydrangia Root, Brigham Tea, Burdock, Black Walnut Hulls, Black Cohosh, Wild Lettuce, Sarsaparilla Root, Valerian and Cayenne. (Editor's note: this product used to contain Chaparral.)

What's it used for? "Helps promote flexibility when used with appropriate diet, exercise and therapy." The key words here are "flexibility" and "therapy." This is an excellent formula for arthritis, bursitis, rheumatism, any condition which limits movement.

Comments: When I broke my toe, I used this to speed recovery. My boyfriend takes it for a sore shoulder, and avoided cortisone shots because of it. Yucca contains natural steroids which reduce inflammation and help rebuild damaged tissue. Black Walnut Hulls kill parasites and help detoxify. Valerian relaxes tense muscles. The other herbs are used in fighting arthritis and similar ailments. A very effective formula, the addition of Cayenne makes it all the more effective.

Summary

Those are some of the most popular products available from Nature's Way. You'll find similar combinations from different companies and

I urge you to look around. You can often find a cheaper brand that has the combination you want. I've chosen Nature's Way because they are the most commonly available herbal products.

———————————— ❧ ————————————

*U*NDERSTANDING THE *N*EW *A*LPHA *H*YDROXY *A*CIDS

By Kelly Quinn

*Y*ou see them everywhere, the newest development in skin care: alpha hydroxy acids or AHA's for short. AHA are fruit acids which are combined in skin care products like moisturizers, make-up and even some tanning products. The idea is a variation on the chemical peelthe acids make the skin shed the top layer faster than exfoliating, revealing newer, younger-looking skin.

Does it work? Many people have noticed an improvement in their complexion after using AHA's. I've tried them but have a hard time remembering to use them regularly, so can't say I've noticed any difference. If you're inclined to try them, there are some things you should know to make your shopping easier.

AHA's generally cause less skin irritation than prescription Retin-A products. Retin-A also causes peeling, but in a more dramatic fashion. Also, when using Retin-A, you should stay out of the sun and use a sun block. AHA's don't require any special preparation, other than clean, dry skin. While AHA's don't usually cause skin irritation, stinging may occur. Some users notice an increase in blemishes for the first few weeks of use as toxins are brought to the surface of the skin.

People with sensitive skin should look for products with the minimal 4% concentration of AHA's. The concentration isn't always stated on the package. Look for the contents to be listed in decreasing order of concentration. Manufacturers suggest looking for a product that has a fruit acid as one of the top four ingredients.

Take a look at what else is in the product. The overall effectiveness can hinge on other non-AHA ingredients as well as the pH level. If the product contains ingredients you usually avoid, the fact that it contains AHA's isn't going to do you much good.

Some products contain ingredients that sound like AHA's, but are not. The Revlon line, for example, contains a neutral molecule, rather than an acidic one. If you're shopping for AHA's at the drugstore or grocery store, rather than a department store, beware products that look like they are AHA products, but don't contain alpha-hydroxy acid at all. Hydroxy Acid Formula is a product that's a good example. It contains salicylic acid.

When trying something new, it's a good idea to research it by going to the cosmetic department of a department store. You don't have to buy there, but the cosmeticians usually are trained in their products and can give excellent advice about what type of AHA would be the best for your skin type. Many will allow you to return products if you are not completely satisfied. Be sure and ask about your store's return policy before buying.

When you know what you want, you can often find comparable products at the drugstore, for much less than department stores. You won't get the service of a department store and the return policy may be more stringent, but you may save enough to make it worth the gamble.

It usually takes about ten days to see any improvement in your complexion, sometimes more. AHA's should be applied morning and evening. If irritation develops, cut it down to once a day and increase gradually. AHA's are not supposed to take the place of a good skin-care routine, but those who have seen results can't say enough about the products and their place in a skin-care regimen.

Using an AHA product won't take the place of a moisturizer, in fact, you may find you need a moisturizer more than ever when using them. Some moisturizers contain AHA's, so once again, read the label.

Recently, the FDA has become interested in AHA's, probably because they are so popular and a gold mine for cosmetic companies. Thus far, there haven't been enough consumer complaints to warrant regulation. But they are under scrutiny. The AHA products available over the counter contain a maximum of 8% to 12% AHA. Anything stronger requires a prescription.

Most products won't tell you the exact percentage of AHA concentration in them, but if you look at the list of ingredients, you can get an idea of which products contain the most of the active ingredient. By law, labels must state the contents in decreasing order of concentration. The AHA's you're most likely to see on the labels are glycolic, lactic, malic, tartaric or citric acids. Less common, but effective nonetheless: pyruvic acid, benzilic acid and mandelic acid.

If you're already on Retin-A, consult with a doctor or pharmacist before using AHA products. AHA's have not been tested on those using Retin-A, so monitoring is essential.

There are now AHA products for all the skin on your body. AHA's are even showing up in some self-tanners, but unless you've been using them regularly on the skin you wish to tan, you won't notice much of a difference in your tan, or your skin. Better to save your money (self-tanners with AHA's are extremely expensive when compared with other brands of self-tanners not containing AHA's) and go with a good quality self-tanner without the AHA additives.

Some AHA products now contain antioxidants. Vitamins A, C, D and E, beta-carotene and superoxide-dismutase. The idea is that the benefits of these free-radical scavengers can promote internal, as well as external benefits when applied to the skin. How much benefit is purely speculative at this point, but it is indeed possible to absorb things into the bloodstream through the skin. Nicotine patches being one example. I wouldn't seek out products containing these ingredients, but if they were in the product I chose, I'd figure it couldn't hurt and might help.

When you go to purchase an AHA product, you may be amazed at all the specialized products. There are AHA gels, creams, night creams, day creams, sunscreens, lip creams, body lotions, the list goes on and on. Rather than buying an entire regime, I suggest you purchase one product, a basic cream or gel and see how you like it before investing a lot of time and money.

Remember, when it comes to looking young, the best bullet to have in your bandolier is free and draws people to you like a magnet: a smile.

WHAT AHA's DO FOR YOUR SKIN

Conventional Exfoliants get rid of dead skin cells by smashing them up one by one to dismantle the top layer.

AHA's dissolve the "glue" between the cells, allowing them to gently float away uncovering smoother, more youthful-looking skin.

SNORING NOT SOMETHING TO TAKE LYING DOWN

By Kelly Quinn

My Dad is the loudest snorer I've ever heard. It was a thing of awe when I was a kid. You could hear him through the closed door and down a flight of stairs. I could never figure out how Mom got any sleep.

I've been told (erroneously, of course) I snore too, sometimes. It's not surprising, as many as 15 percent of women and 25 percent of men are habitual snorers. Thirty percent of women and forty percent of men snore intermittently.

Many factors contribute to snoring, even age can make a difference. Once you get past age 60 your chances of being a snorer go up to 40 percent for women and 60 percent for men. Virtually everyone snores sometimes, but there are times when snoring can indicate a serious, potentially life-threatening situation.

The most significant possibility is that the snoring signals the presence of obstructive sleep apnea, a dangerous disorder in which the snorer actually stops breathing, sometimes hundreds of times during the night. As many as half of those who snore probably have some degree of apnea, according to the experts.

Apnea is a dangerous condition because the interruption in breathing lowers oxygen levels in the blood, which has been linked to blood pressure problems, strokes and heart attacks.

Even if the snorer isn't suffering from apnea there are potential health risks. Snorers tend to wake several times a night and often get up in the morning exhausted. Why do people snore? Snoring is a noise made by the vibration of soft parts of the upper airway, usually caused when something partially obstructs the airway.

So what do you do if you or someone you sleep with snores? Basically, there are three categories of potential solutions to the problem.

The easiest to try and the least extreme or expensive solutions are those in the lifestyle category. Making some changes in your life could end the problem. If you are overweight, shed some pounds. Sleep on a pillow that lifts your chin as far away from your chest as possible. Don't drink alcohol anywhere near bedtime. Sew a tennis ball in the back of the snorer's pajamas. Get earplugs or turn on some "white noise," like a fan.

The next category contains the more unusual, expensive and bizarre remedies. A device that sells for $59 straps onto the wrist and gives the wearer a mild electric shock, awakening him every time he snores. You can buy the Breathe Right Nasal Dilator in ten-packs for about $6 a pack. It's a disposable adhesive strip that goes over the bridge of the nose to hold the nostrils open, supposedly increasing nasal breathing by 30 percent. More expensive, but pretty well proven is the CPAP (Continuous Positive Airway Pressure) mask, which is the first line of treatment for both apnea and snoring. It's a mask, fitting over the nose and connected to a small fan, that you wear at night. It pushes air through to the back of the throat.

The last resort is surgery. Tonsillectomies can solve the problem if tonsils are very large and protrude into the airway. Other forms of surgery are also used to remove obstructionseven laser surgery is being used. In laser surgery, the patient makes several trips to a doctor's office to trim small amounts each time from the soft palate and the uvula. Less painful that other surgical methods, it is considered effective for snoring, but has not been tested extensively for apnea.

For most of us, snoring is little more than an annoying inconvenience. But if you snore and aren't feeling rested in the morning, it's a good idea to see your doctor. If all you'd like is a good night's uninterrupted sleep, but the noise keeps you awake, try a relaxing herb, like Valerian. Chamomile tea before bedtime can be good for restful sleep. Make sure the room is properly humidified as dryness can cause snoring.

Sleep well.

Dear Reader,

About 10 years ago, I had an idea for a story. It went like this:

Washington, DC—At a little past noon on a Wednesday, two men park a Volkswagen van on the top floor of a parking ramp near the Capitol. They leave the ramp, walk a block and get on a city bus.

Two hours later, at 2:30 on that Wednesday afternoon, the nuclear bomb in the Volkswagen van detonates and much of Washington DC. is vaporized. Chaos ensues.

I didn't write the story because I thought it would happen. I still think it will—now more than ever. So many people hate us and there are so many nuclear bombs available for sale sooner or later, anyone who wants to buy one, will. And he won't need a rocket to deliver it.

Let's hope and pray it never happens, but be prepared.

Some herbs protect us against radiation by blocking the absorption of radioactive isotopes, cheating isotopes from our bodies and minimizing damage. At Hiroshima, the Japanese discovered a diet of mismo protects against radiation.

The pectin in raw Sunflower Seeds binds radioactive strontium in the intestines to reduce absorption into the bones. Kelp removes strontium 90 from the body and prevents absorption of radioactive iodine, which causes thyroid cancer in children. Cayenne works in the liver to block carcinogens. Aloe Vera removes dead skin from radiation burns and feeds the living tissue. Milk Thistle is essential to protect the liver.

Nutritionists also recommend Algin, Vitamins A, E, C, B-B-Complex and F, Pantothenic Acid and Brewer's Yeast.

The most effective protective herb of all, according to many herbalists and researchers, is Siberian Ginseng, also called Eluthero. It protects, heals, stimulates and regenerates cells.

It's good to know how to protect yourself—especially since your doctor doesn't. There is so much ambient radiation these days, we don't need another disaster to put ourselves at risk.

Be sure to take these protective herbs before X-rays. Siberian Ginseng also protects against chemotherapy and speeds recover, but let's hope that never happens to you, either.

Take care of yourself,

*F*IND THE *R*IGHT *S*PECIALTY *P*RODUCT FOR *M*EN & *W*OMEN

By Kelly Quinn

*T*oo often, we get up our courage to try something new only to discover upon entering a health food store that we can't find what we want. The clerks may not know much about the product you're seeking, other than if they can reorder it for you.

To make the health food store not so ominous, we will focus on the most popular formulas on the market: the Nature's Way product line of herbal formulas. Nature's Way makes many other products as well, most of them predominantly placed in your local health store. Even some main-stream drugstores carry them, now.

We will explore Nature's Way's line of specialty products for men and women. Use this as a reference when looking at other comparable products, of which there are many. We use the Nature's Way products as examples and they are among the easiest products to find. However, there are other manufacturers out there that make similar formulas with quality ingredients for what may cost less.

MEN'S PRODUCT LINE

Ginsun *(Panax extract)*: "Ginsun is a concentrated Korean Panax ginseng extract standardized to 7% ginsenosides" according to product literature. Whatever that means—I must confess I don't know and I don't really want to find out. You probably don't want to know either. The literature goes on and on about their state-of-the-art process for extraction and premium ginseng.

What's it used for? To provide energy and the other many beneficial effects of ginseng: improve immune system, enhance sex drive, improve all-around performance.

Comments: I wouldn't recommend this product or any other containing ginseng extracts of any kind. Most ginseng has the potential to increase heart rate and provide a general feeling of anxiousness — feeling wired. If whole ginseng is taken, rather than an extract, the risk of side-effects is lower, the benefits higher. If you want to take ginseng, good for you! But try to get it in an herbal formula. There are some with Sarsaparilla, Fo-Ti, Gotu Kola and Saw Palmetto Berries, like Nature's Way's own APH Formula. Or even get a bottle of the whole herb, powdered ginseng.

Co Q10 *(Coenzyme Q10):* This is one of the hot new supplements, claimed to cure everything from asthma to cancer. While it has gotten a lot of attention for many years in Japan, only recently did interest surface in this country. Product information is extremely slim, only detailing the size of the capsules. Apparently, Nature's Way isn't too sure about this one either.

What's it used for? A supplement that is expensive and some say needless, it has shown benefits as far as improving general well-being and overall health. Lot's of hype about this one, little solid information.

Comments: I'd pass on this one, too. You can get proven benefits, much cheaper using Cayenne.

Omega 3 Fish Oils: A nutritional supplement of polyunsaturated Omega 3 series fish oil containing 18% EPA and 12% DHA. Made of Marine fish oils, natural vitamin E.

What's it used for? For those who are into fish oils, it can lower cholesterol, decrease the risk of coronary disease among other benefits.

Comments: I don't really know anyone who is into fish oils anymore, but if you are, this looks to be a quality product that delivers the goods.

Proactive: Standardized extract of Saw Palmetto Berries. Recommended use by men over the age of 50.

What's it used for? Saw Palmetto Berries are widely known as a treatment for the glands, including the prostate. It is thought they may help avoid and possibly treat prostate cancer. It is also thought to be useful in regaining sex drive in men.

Comments: If I were taking this for all-over good health, I'd prefer to take whole herbs, perhaps an herbal combination with some other herbs like Sarsaparilla, Damiana, Ginseng. The herbs synergize together and can provide greater benefit. If, however, I was dealing with cancer or a pre-cancerous condition, an extract would be acceptable.

Sarsaparilla: A tropical herb from Central America.

What's it used for? According to the product literature, "A tonic herb popular with athletes." So, that means we'll get energy from it. It is also used in sexual rejuvenation-balancing formulas as it feeds the adrenals.

Comments: This is a good herb for both men and women to take. Preferably as part of one of the herbal combinations mentioned above.

PR Formula: Contains Cayenne, Uva Ursi Leaves, Parsley, Golden-seal Root, Gravel Root, Juniper Berries, Marshmallow Root, Ginger Root and Siberian Ginseng Root. "Popular with men over 50" is the key phrase in the product literature. Think about what happens in men over 50.

What's it used for? This formula should give energy, help cut the risk of heart disease and also has herbs for the prostate and urinary system. It could improve sex drive, too.

Comments: The only herb I have a problem with is Goldenseal which should be used only for infections. However, the other herbs in this formula are so perfect for men, particularly those over 50, that I'd have to recommend this product.

H Formula: Contains Hawthorne Berries, Cayenne, Vitamin E and Lecithin.

What's it used for? No clues in the product literature, but I'd assume it's used as a formula to prevent heart disease and give energy.

Comments: All the ingredients in this formula synergize well together and make for an effective formula for overall health.

B/P Formula: Contains Cayenne, Parsley, Ginger Root, Goldenseal Root, Garlic Clove and Siberian Ginseng Root.

What's it used for? Product literature says it's used to promote general good health and especially used for circulation and physical fitness. You'd use this product as a cardiovascular stimulant, a heart disease preventative, a source of natural energy.

Comments: I have a problem with the inclusion of Goldenseal and would suggest you look for another product without it. Parsley is a natural diuretic and could be helpful if there is any tendency toward fluid retention, however it is really not a very significant player in this formula. If you're already taking a product with Siberian Ginseng, taking this product would increase your dosage, possibly making you feel wired. Otherwise, this would be a good product to take.

SPECIALTY PRODUCTS FOR WOMEN

Cantrol: Contains anti-oxidant capsules, lactobacillus acidophilus supplement, caprylic acid, linseed oil and Pau d'Arco.

What's it used for? Product literature goes on and on about how it fits into a nutritional support program, but nothing really specific. I'd assume it was for those prone to yeast infections and bladder infections.

Comments: This product could be useful in those who suffer chronic yeast or bladder infections. It would also be a good choice if you're undergoing treatment with antibiotics, to prevent such infections. As a part of a daily program with no risk factors however, I don't think this is necessary. Eat yogurt every day instead and save your money.

Caprinex *(Caprylic Acid):* I have to admit I'd never heard of Caprylic Acid before but the product literature tells us it is a fatty acid found in coconuts and other foods, and produced in small amounts by the body. Why we'd want to take it is a mystery.

What's it used for? You got me. But I'd guess it's yet another nutritional support method.

Comments: If intrigued, I'd be inclined to try a bottle and see if I noticed a difference. If not, I'd blow this one off.

Change-O-Life Formula: Contains Black Cohosh Root, Sarsaparilla Root, Siberian Ginseng Root, Licorice, Blessed Thistle, Squawvine and False Unicorn Root.

What's it used for? This is a good formula for women undergoing menopause and those with PMS or menstrual-related difficulties, including low sex drive. Black Cohosh is a hormone regulating herb, Sarsaparilla, Siberian Ginseng and Licorice provide energy and are particularly useful for women. Caution, Licorice can raise blood pressure, so keep an eye on yourself. Ginseng and Licorice can make some people feel wired. Blessed Thistle, Squawvine and False Unicorn Root are all very effective as uterine toners, useful in eliminating cramps, excess fluid and mood swings.

Comments: I've taken this product, although I'm nowhere near the "change-o-life" yet. It was helpful in relieving PMS and painful menstruation. I take a product like this every day.

FemCal: Is a calcium supplement that features the high bioavailability of calcium citrate.

What's it used for? It's recommended women get 1,000-1,500mg. of calcium daily to prevent osteoporosis.

Comments: If you are interested in taking a calcium supplement, this would be a good one.

Fem-Mend Formula: Contains Goldenseal Root, Blessed Thistle, Cayenne, Uva Ursi, Cramp Bark, False Unicorn Root, Red Raspberry Leaves, Squawvine and Ginger Root.

What's it used for? Product literature says: "A monthly supplement for women." That pretty much says it. All the herbs in this formula are beneficial to women with PMS or painful, unpleasant menstrual cycles.

Comments: I've used this one, but since it contains Goldenseal, I vary it with something similar, but without the Goldenseal. Otherwise, an excellent formula.

Female Select Formula: For those who are into enzymes, Nature's Way has you covered, too. This product also contains a complementary herbal base of Spirulina, Alfa Max Concentrate, Dong Quai Root and Beet Root.

What's it used for? Enzymes, particularly live enzymes are gaining popularity as supplements for good health. The herbs in the product can be helpful in total nutrition and stabilizing hormonal balance, however the amount in the product must be small as it's called "a complementary base."

Comments: If you are going to use herbs to treat female problems, better to find a different formula containing only whole herbs. If you want to try enzymes, this would be a nice, low-key way to start.

These formulas should give you a good start in finding which herbs and supplements work best for you.

WRAP UP SUMMER AND GET BACK TO WORK

By Kelly Quinn

September is the traditional time to pack up our summer toys, put away that swimming suit and cover up our tans with business or back-to-school attire. Sometimes, it's hard to see summer end, looking ahead to another year of drudgery before we can once again relax and bask in the sun.

Fortunately, it doesn't have to be completely miserable. We can't tell you how to extend your time at the beach (weekends!), but we can tell you how to feel better while you figure it all out.

As summer draws to a close, we find we tend to try to cram everything in that we didn't get a chance to do before. That can mean pushing your body more than is wise with too many late nights, too much fun in the sun and not enough sleep. Avoid a late-summer illness by keeping up your health regimen as much as you are able. Maybe you only remembered to take your supplements once yesterday. That's okay, at least you remembered. Maybe you don't have time to work out everyday, besides, you've been at the beach a lot and that's physical right? Try to schedule some workout time every day¡even if it means not working out as long. You need it to keep your body on track and for the mental clarity and emotional lift it brings. Especially if you're busy, you need the break exercise provides—not a nap.

But you may find you catch that cold that's been going around anyway. We've noticed amazing results with the Pleurisy Root Blend SP-3 by Solaray. It runs under $10 for 100 capsules and is just fabulous. It contains **pleurisy root, wild cherry bark, slippery elm bark, plantain, mullein leaves, chickweed, horehound, licorice root, kelp, ginger root** and **saw palmetto berries.**

Pleurisy root, wild cherry bark, slippery elm bark and mullein leaves are effective cough suppressants and calm the bronchial tubes. Horehound, licorice root and ginger root act as expectorants, so the chest stays clearer with less coughing—the coughs are more productive. Kelp, plantain and saw palmetto berries nourish the glands and the entire system and chickweed calms and detoxifies. Chickweed is excellent in the treatment of chronic bronchial problems, particularly those stemming from such variables as poor air quality, allergies, etc. It's also high in vitamin C.

Put all these herbs together and you get a product that truly works like gangbusters. A young friend of mine, Michelle, had been on preventative asthma medication and cough syrup. She had been coughing a lot and was very congested.

Michelle took four capsules of the pleurisy root blend and within half an hour, we noticed a marked improvement. She stayed on the herbs for the weekend, in addition to the cough syrup. By the end of the weekend, she sounded almost totally back to normal and had stopped taking the asthma medication. She was also able to get off the cough syrup.

While Michelle was taking the herbs, my boyfriend was having house guests. He came upon one of them in the kitchen in the wee hours;she couldn't sleep because she'd been coughing, too. He gave her four capsules of the pleurisy root blend. The next morning, she wanted more. They'd worked!

Our air quality was terrible over the weekend. I noticed myself coughing more in the mornings and evenings. I've been taking the stuff once a day as a preventative and it has indeed worked. It also seems to have a beneficial effect on clearing nasal congestion. Everyone who has tried this stuff has asked for more. Unfortunately, I've found it hard to find. Try to get your health store to order it if they don't normally carry it. Most will be happy to order things, as it means they'll have a regular customer.

I don't know about your family, but mine was totally stressed out, dreading the return to work and school. I dreaded the regimentation and daily grind, the kids were panicked about making new friends and doing all that homework again. They started complaining about not being able to sleep, about their faces breaking out and being constantly on edge.

So, I put them on **gotu kola** and **valerian**. The gotu kola de-stresses them, gives them natural energy, detoxifies them and gives them glowing, clear skin. They take three capsules, two times a day.

I'm on it, too.

Valerian helps them sleep. I don't take it because sleep is rarely my problem. They've been taking the NiteCaps line from Heartfoods, but any of the valerian blends on the market would do as well. They take the valerian about an hour before bedtime and seem much better rested upon arising.

Now that we're back to only weekends off, many will try until the snow flies to be active every weekend, playing football, etc. That means a lot of people will be experiencing muscle and back pain. We've got something for that, too.

A friend asked me what to try for his back. It'd been bothering him for quite some time. Steve had been on muscle relaxants and pain pills for awhile, but nothing seemed to do much good. I put him on **valerian, yucca** and **cayenne**. The valerian was to stop the spasms in the muscle—it's a natural muscle relaxant, that's why it's so good for sleep. The yucca contains natural steroids to rebuild and strengthen the muscle.

Cayenne improves circulation, which speeds healing. Certain acids are released when a muscle is injured. That's what causes much of the pain—particularly if the muscle is simply painful due to overuse. When you move and work the muscle, the acids are worked out of it and that's why after awhile, it doesn't hurt as much. This is nature's way of making sure we take it easy when we've overdone it and our bodies need time to heal. Cayenne speeds the process by detoxification. I put him on the 40,000 heat unit cayenne with ginger. He has yet to complain of a pepper attack, but he has commented on how much better he feels. We couldn't be happier!

When illness threatens, heavy up a little on the supplements you are taking. If you normally take herbs, increase the immune system builders and germ fighters. Go heavy on the **garlic, cayenne, gotu kola, ashwagandhi** and **vitamin C**. Try to get more rest. Exercise, but don't overtax yourself. Try to eat a little more than usual, at least don't skip meals. Try to get more fruits and vegetables into your diet. My sister swears that eating a lemon wipes out a cold. My Dad tried it and said it worked for him. I find that a dragon cocktail of cayenne/garlic blend pepper mixed with V8 or tomato juice knocks out any cold at the first sign of one.

Keep an eye on yourself. Act at the first sign of illness and you'll likely have a happy, healthy autumn.

OUR FAVORITE HERBS: GOTU KOLA

By Kelly Quinn

Anyone who's used or tried to use herbs knows one thing for sure: there are a lot of herbs. Hundreds, maybe even thousands. How do you remember what to use for what? Where do you even start?

What makes an herb one of our favorites? The ones that are good for a multitude of uses, as opposed to one specific application, usually win hands down. These are the herbs you'll want to make sure you take or at least store in your medicine chest. They are the herbs you'll probably need for yourself or someone else.

Gotu kola is one of those herbs from which anyone could benefit. A common plant in India, Pakistan, Malaysia and areas in Eastern Europe, it's a circulatory herb, used to treat diseases of the skin, blood and nervous system, as well as depression, fever, inflammation and is an anti-aging herb.

Gotu kola is used in Asia and Europe to cool and detoxify the blood by neutralizing blood acids. For centuries, gotu kola has been used to treat leprosy, syphilis, tuberculosis, psoriasis, cervicitis, vaginitis, acne, headaches, blisters and stomach aches. According to Shannon Quinn in *Left For Dead,* gotu kola contains four major constituents which aid the function of the immune system by partially breaking down the walls of diseased cells, making the microbes easier to kill. It also speeds the healing of wounds by stimulating cell division. Volatile oils in the herb have a diuretic and blood purifying property and help lower serum cholesterol levels. Flavonoids in the herb help control spasms in muscles. Gotu kola displays a wide range of antibiotic activity and can be used as an antibacterial, antifungal, antiameobic and insecticidal agent.

The medicinal part of the plant is the top. The dried leaves can be brewed as a tea or taken in capsule form. According to *Left For Dead*, make the tea using 1 ounce of herb for each pint of water. The usual dose is 3 ounces of tea, three times a day, or 5 to 10 capsules three times a day.

Gotu kola oil can be applied over the entire body, including the scalp to treat nervous disorders. To make the oil, cover 1 part powdered leaves with 3 parts sesame oil. Let stand covered, one to 14 days, then filter. I would imagine Grape seed oil or other light, natural oils would work as well as dried leaves as opposed to powdered.

How would gotu kola fit into your life? If you are under stress (and who isn't?), gotu kola can help, not as a relaxant, but as an energizer. You handle the stress because you have more energy, more strength to deal with life. That's how gotu kola affected me.

My boyfriend's son had a lot of things going on in his life. He was going to be living with his dad, starting a new school, making new friends and adopting a new lifestyle. Matthew was excited and looking forward to all the new things, but there was still an element of stress.

About a week before school started, Matt's parents noticed he'd developed a twitch. Figuring it was due to stress, Matt started taking gotu kola in the morning and afternoon. His tic disappeared and he's doing very well in school, enjoying life immensely.

I put my daughter on it to prepare her for school and quell an outbreak of teenage acne. She's doing great and her skin has improved tremendously.

When I started taking gotu kola, my skin was broken out, I was overweight, tired, stressed and headachy all the time. Life sucked. But after a couple weeks on the stuff (I made a tea and drank 32 ounces a day), I was exercising with genuine pleasure, my skin had cleared up and I felt I could handle life¡and I did.

I've also taken gotu kola when I've had one of those late-day headaches and was delighted to find relief within twenty minutes.

Gotu kola is also good for the cardio-vascular system, acting as a toner and stimulant. I've been unable to find any contraindications for gotu kola, nor any indication that it's possible to overdose. I would be more concerned about underdosing. I would give it to both children and adults as a strengthening, anti-aging herb that can help assure they'll be at their best every day.

All these reasons and more make gotu kola one of our favorite herbs. Try it and I'm sure it will become one of yours, too.

ℋELP 𝒴OURSELF
𝒞HOOSE A ℒAXATIVE

By Kelly Quinn

𝒩o matter who you are, at some point, you are going to find yourself looking for a product to give nature a little kick in the behind, if you know what I mean. While there are many laxative-type products over-the-counter in pharmacies, they have a tendency to cause gas, bloating, cramps and diarrhea. Overuse of laxatives can result in a laxative-dependence. Most of the over-the-counter variety contain mineral oils and/or fiber to get things moving. Fortunately, there are natural products which do the trick with few of the side-effects or hazards.

How do you know if you need a laxative? It's not as simple as it sounds. If you experience abdominal pain, gas or bloating, you may want to try a natural laxative to ensure the system is indeed being properly cleansed. Keep that in mind for children, too.

Once my daughter had horrendous abdominal pain. I called the doctor, fearful of appendicitis (I can never remember which side the thing is on). We'd been experiencing a Santa Ana condition (high, dry winds and extreme heat) and the doctor told me to give her 16 ounces of warm water and some Milk of Magnesia. He said he doubted she'd been getting enough fluids in the past couple of days and to tank up on liquids.

We took his advice and he was right. My daughter felt much better within hours. Now that's the first thing I think of when one of the kids complains about abdominal pain. Even if the person has had a bowel movement, according to my doctor, it might not be complete.

Another way to tell if you need a laxative is if your schedule gets thrown off or you notice you aren't needing the bathroom as frequently these days. Travel, stress, a change in habits, all can trigger constipation.

The first thing to do if the constipation is due to a schedule or lifestyle change is to give your body a chance to do what it has to do. Don't go for the laxatives immediately. It's okay to have some variation in bathroom habits. Drink a lot of water, go heavy on the fruits and vegetables¡it's true what they say about prune juice! Eat something fat-laden (a White Castle hamburger has been known to cure many a case!).

There are basically two types of laxatives. A "bulk-forming" laxative is a fiber product that adds bulk and retains water to ease elimination. A "stimulant" laxative is one that stimulates the normal contractions of the bowel. Most over-the-counter laxatives contain fiber and/or mineral oils to get things moving, along with some chemical drugs. Mineral oil is used as a stool-softener, which is why when relief comes, it often comes in the form of diarrhea.

Some people swear by assorted enemas and high colonics, but there are some things I must admit I have no desire to try. I would always much prefer taking a drink of something or a capsule, or eating a different food, to hauling out equipment or having to go to a special place that gives high-powered enemas. I also have no desire to scour my colon and find all sorts of disgusting things were in there, as some touters of special cleansing products expouse. No, I just want to feel good and know that my system is working the way it should without any major leaps in technology.

That's what's great about herbs. No muss, no fuss, your body is back on track and you don't have to feel anything less than wonderful if you don't want to. They're safe for everyone. *(Of course, pregnant women should check with their health-care practitioner before taking any laxative or diuretic products.)*

Aloe Vera juice is one of the gentlest laxatives around. It's a multiuse herb, one worth keeping on hand at all times. Not only does it gently cleanse the system, it's something that you can drink every day. If you have liver, kidney or other gastrointestinal ills, many herbalists recommend you drink at least an ounce of Aloe Juice daily.

Aloe is also good for upset and nervous stomachs. It does not cause diarrhea or cramping. You just notice that things work. I suggest the Aloe that is cold-pressed, with active enzymes. You can buy Aloe Juice flavored, or plain. Plain Aloe doesn't taste bad, it just doesn't taste good, either. I suggest if you don't find the taste palatable, try adding 1 part Aloe to 1 part soda (7up or Ginger ale type soda, basically anything but Cola, which can irritate the stomach) or 1 part juice. I find the unflavored Aloe seems to work better in smaller amounts than the flavored version.

Other herbs you can use to combat constipation include (you can try these either singly or look for them as part of an herbal formula): barberry, cayenne, dandelion root, mandrake, psyllium, turkey rhubarb, fennel and cascara sagrada. All work gently and subtly, so you don't spend all your time hanging out near bathrooms.

The excellent book of herbal formulas *Herbally Yours,* by Penny C. Royal, lists herbs for formulating a colon healing and cleansing formula:

Alfalfa	Chlorophyll	Myrrh
Aloe Vera*	Comfrey	Psyllium*
Barberry	Fenugreek	Slippery Elm*
Bayberry	Eucalyptus	Strawberry
Cascara Sagrada*	Ginger	Taheebo
Chamomile	Hyssop	Turkey Rhubarb
Chickweed	Mullein	Yarrow

*Particularly effective.

Cascara sagrada will improve bowel tone and bring about a permanent beneficial effect. **Fenugreek** helps to lubricate the colon. **Hyssop** and **mullein** are good for decreasing mucous. To help heal the colon, use 1/2 cup distilled water, 1 tablespoon Cider vinegar, 1 teaspoon honey and 1/4 teaspoon cayenne several times a day.

Herbally Yours also recommends the following herbs when making a formula for constipation:

Aloe Vera	Couch Grass	Mullein
Barberry	Dandelion	Poke Weed
Blessed Thistle	Ginseng	Psyllium
Buckthorn	Goldenseal	Red Raspberry
Cascara Sagrada	Licorice	Slippery Elm
Chickweed	Mandrake	Turkey Rhubarb

Aloe Vera is used internally 1 ounce 4 to 5 times a day. It is especially good for chronic constipation in older people.

If you're not inclined to make a formula yourself, you can try one of the following products available at your local health store, or one similar:

Aloelax by Nature's Way contains aloe ferox and fennel seed. Aloe ferox, according to the product literature is one of the strongest natural laxatives known, and fennel seed relaxes the intestines to reduce cramping. Recommended only for severe or stubborn constipation. Not recommended for children, the elderly or pregnant women.

Aloe Vera from Nature's Way is an herbal laxative that works to cleanse the large intestine. Nature's Way doesn't recommend it for children, the elderly or during pregnancy, but to be honest, I'd try it if I were a kid or elderly. Nature's Way is trying to protect itself with the warning, but Aloe is one of the safest laxatives known to man.

FiberCleanse from Nature's Way is a bulk-forming laxative. Product literature recommends the product for those with sensitive systems or mild constipation. Contains psyllium, fennel seed and bentonite. Available in bulk powder and in capsules. Safe for kids, the elderly and pregnant women. However, the fiber could cause cramping and bloating and I have never heard of bentonite. I would probably try a different product before this one. If you use this, be sure to drink plenty of water¡at least 20 ounces.

Naturalax #1 Formula by Nature's Way contains psyllium husks and senna leaves. It provides bulk fiber and a stimulant laxative in capsule form. Referred to as gentle strength. This would be a good product to try.

Naturalax #2 Formula, also by Nature's Way, is listed as medium strength. It contains cascara sagrada bark, barberry root bark, fennel seed, ginger root, goldenseal root, lobelia herb, red raspberry leaves, turkey rhubarb foot and cayenne. The original herbal formula from Dr. John Christopher and their most popular laxative formula. With good reason, as it truly is an excellent formula.

Naturalax #3 Formula is referred to as extra strength by Nature's Way. It contains: aloe, cascara sagrada bark, butternut bark, fennel seed, ginger root, red raspberry leaves and peppermint leaves. recommended for relief of occasional irregularity, the product promises results in 6 to 12 hours. A good formula.

If you can find a formula similar to those listed above, it should work as well as the Nature's Way brand. We use Nature's Way as product examples simply because they are by far the most popular and easiest to obtain.

Don't forget to try remedies you might have around the house before you go out and buy something. Sometimes just eating a few apples or some vegetables and drinking a lot of water will do the trick. With all the herbal remedies, you should have no problem helping yourself feel great.

TREATMENTS FOR VARICOSE VEINS

By Dick Quinn

Varicose veins are a maddening problem. They effect appearance, often entail painful bulging and could presage life-threatening clots.

Conventional allopathic treatments employ surgery and injection.

"Compression injection" involves the injection of a hardening agent to block and deaden the vein, so the body absorbs it and forms new circulatory channels.

The "compression injection" method is very popular in Europe. It is less expensive, less intrusive, and can be less painful than surgery, but it has a failure rate up to 45%. It often leaves stains on the skin and can result in phlebitis, infection, and other complication.

Surgery has its expense and danger, too. Surgery may not make your legs look better, either. "Stripping" is a procedure where a rod is inserted in the vein at the ankle and run through it to the groin. The vein is then severed at the top and the rod is withdrawn, pulling the vein out with it.

In America, varicose veins affect about 25% of the women and 10% of the men. Up to 50% of adult Europeans have them, but only 2% of the women of Africa and India.

There are many theories about causes, but varicose veins result from poor circulation to the heart, which raises pressure in veins in the leg. Blood is trapped in the legs when faulty valves in veins leading to the heart leak, permitting blood to drain back into the leg between heartbeats.

The condition is often associated with pregnancy or obesity. Some say it's hereditary; others that it has behavioral or nutritional causes. Constipation is said to be a causative factor, because it leads to "straining at the stool," which increases blood pressure in the legs. There is little agreement on any single cause, but all agree, the best treatment is prevention.

Here are simple suggestions from allopathic and holistic practitioners:
• Sit and stand a little as possible. When walking, the powerful muscles of the calf and thigh act like a "second heart," pumping the blood up, out of the leg. Walking can lower leg veinal blood pressure 30%.
• Exercise your legs often to strengthen calf muscles.
• Whenever possible, raise your feet higher than your heart. Lay on your back on the floor and put your feet up against the wall or on a chair. Relax. Breathe deeply. Let go. Ah-h-h-h.
• Go barefoot, wear sandals, or flat shoes.
• Do not drink aloe—it draws blood to the legs.
• No hot baths, hot soaks, or hot pads on your legs (end each shower by splashing cold water on them.
• Cross your legs less often (it restricts circulation).
• Avoid hard chairs; sitting restricts circulation.
• Avoid flour, sugar, and other simple carbohydrates. Stop smoking (damages veins), eat parsley often and diet, if overweight. If your blood pressure is high, take valerian, garlic, and cayenne; diet and exercise to lower it.

Herbs to treat varicose veins
• For leg pain, take 400 i.u. of Vitamin E with every meal (1,200 daily).
• To boost peripheral circulation, especially in the legs, use cayenne, ginger, and prickly ash bark. Rue is also recommended, but must not be used when pregnant. (If pregnant, drink parsley and oatstraw tea to strengthen veins; and nettle tea for veinal elasticity.)
• To strengthen veins, take butcher's broom, hawthorn, buckwheat, and bilberry extract. Horse chestnuts are recommended, but hard to obtain and must be shelled, soaked, boiled 1/2 hour, and ground before eating.
• To control water retention, use yarrow and dandelion leaves.

Topical: aloe vera juice; tea made from witch hazel leaves, and calendula (marigold) flowers, white oak bark, and wintergreen oil. Boil comfrey root and use cooked root and its tea as a poultice on problem veins.

Other herbs to treat varicose veins include bayberry and pau de arco in tea or capsules.
Good luck!

Shingles:
Some Answers to
a Painful Problem

By Dick Quinn

If you have not yet had shingles, you may not know what it's like to be truly miserable. But be warned; if you had chicken pox as a child, you're at risk of shingles as an adult.

Herpes Zoster (shingles) is a viral infection that follows nerves in your chest, neck, lower back, forehead , and face, causing painful burning, itching blisters. The pain can be severe and the condition can last for weeks (even months. Shingles are most severe if you are over 40. The pain is constant, precluding sleep and normal activity.

The root cause is the varicella zoster (VZ) virus, which is left alive in the body after recovery from chicken pox. The VZ virus is held in check by the immune system until an illness, injury, or other trauma causes it to be released into the nerves. It is not contagious.

The most powerful and most effective shingles painkiller is **Cayenne**. It's available in a salve called Zostrix, which is an expensive prescription preparation. You can also make your own cayenne salve using either ground cayenne or capsaicin extract from the health store, mixed into a calendula (marigold) or other type of healing herbal salve. For maximum healing effect, add some liquid **vitamin E** to the salve or apply it to the blisters separately.

Cayenne does not damage tissue, so you can apply as much as you want as often as needed. It will kill the pain and promote healing.

Even after the blisters heal, the aching "posttherpetic" pain can last for years. This deep pain has been effectively treated with **vitamin C** (500 to 1,000 mg. per hour) and **vitamin E** in capsules (1,200 − 1,600 I.U. daily with meals).

Acupuncture has been effective in relieving pain, slowing the spread of the rash and healing the blisters. In research conducted in California by Dr. Nolan Cordon, 10 of 11 patients treated with acupuncture found the intense pain was controlled and healing promoted. **Note: Do not take Tylenol or other painkillers containing acetaminophen** (they will prolongand worsen the pain and illness.

The amino acid **L-lysine**, available at any heath store, is thought to diminish the severity and combat the spread of Herpes virus illnesses including shingles. The recommended dosage is 500 mg. twice daily; also **B complex**, 100 mg. 3 times daily, helps damaged nerves heal.

Aloe vera has also proved to alleviate pain and promote healing. Split the leaf and apply the soft gelatin to blisters and sores. Tea made with the herb plantain can be drunk or used topically to treat shingles.

Herbs for shingles are formulated to attack the VZ virus, stop the spread, heal the blisters, cleanse the lower bowel, remove toxins from the blood, correct hormonal balance, provide sustaining energy and heal the body.

HERBAL FORMULA TO BE TAKEN IN CAPSULES OR IN JUICE:

Shingles Formula 3 parts Chaparral (attacks the virus, free radicals, and tumors)

2 parts Manjhista (if this anti-herpes herb from India is unavailable, substitute English Madder)

1 part Cayenne mixed with…

   1/2 part Turmeric

   1 part Yarrow (flowers, ground; a blood cleaner)

   1 part Dandelion Root (cleanses lower bowel)

   1 part Chinese Licorice (hormonal; energy)

   1 part granulated Garlic mixed with

      1/2 part granulated Onion for synergy

   1 part Myrrh with 1/2 part Goldenseal (anti viral/anti bacterial)

Blend and encapsulate or store in airless glass jar in refrigerator. It can be eaten with food, mixed into juice, or in capsules. Take 12-20 capsules (6 to 10 grams; a level to rounded teaspoon) or more daily before meals. Adjust the dose according to need. There is no overdose danger since none of these herbs are toxic.

Other safe herbs that could be included in our formula include **black walnut leaves** *(anti-viral),* **yucca** *(causes body to make cortisone),* kelp *(mineral balance)*, red clover *(cleaning, anti-tumor)*, yellow dock *(glandular cleanser)*, comfrey *(healing)*, wheat grass *(chlorophyll)*, skullcap *(neurological)*, and hawthorn *(cleansing, heart energy)*.

Taken on food, as tea or in capsules, each has been used effectively to combat shingles.

I'm a candidate for the shingles virus, too. If it attacks me, I intend to throw everything at it. I hope this gives you some new ways to protect yourself.

$\mathcal{H}$ELP $\mathcal{Y}$OURSELF $\mathcal{F}$IND THE $\mathcal{P}$RODUCT $\mathcal{Y}$OU $\mathcal{W}$ANT

By Kelly Quinn

*A*vailable in many health stores coast-to-coast, the products can also be ordered by calling 1-800-CAYENNE. Originally founded by Dick Quinn, author of *Left For Dead* and publisher of this publication, Heartfoods uses many of the original Dick Quinn formulas. The product line has expanded so we'll review their entire line of formulas.

Cayenne Power Plus! Caps: Product literature calls this the "ultimate power experience" with over 130,000 heat units (h.u.) of African Birdseye Cayenne. It also contains Ginger. Although Heartfoods says the product is not for first-time Cayenne users, I can't recommend this product for anyone. For the most part, the hotter the Cayenne the better, but when you reach such high heat units¡over 100,000 or so, the Cayenne starts to work against you, negating many of the benefits. Users of this product have complained of feeling tired, drained and all-around malaise. Far better to use a Cayenne product under 105,000 h.u. and take more if you still don't feel the energy.

Cayenne Power Caps: The original Dick Quinn formula, contains 100,000 h.u. Cayenne, Ginger, Hawthorn Berries and Lecithin. This is a good product for anyone needing the benefits of Cayenne. The Ginger eases it into your system and enhances the benefits of the Cayenne. Hawthorn Berries repair the heart muscle and strengthen the heart. Lecithin is used to prevent the Cayenne burn and provides many ancillary benefits.

Cayenne Heart Food Caps: Another original Dick Quinn formula, this is what my family and I take. It contains 100,000 h.u. Cayenne, Garlic, Hawthorn Berries, Onion, Ginger and Lecithin. This product provides the benefits of Power Caps, but also the additional benefits of Garlic (fights high blood pressure, natural antibiotic, synergizes with the Cayenne) and Onion (a natural infection-fighter, Onion prevents Garlic body odor).

Cayenne Health Food Caps: Are just right for people who'd sure like to take Cayenne but are either afraid or can't tolerate it. I've never heard of anyone experiencing a Cayenne burn with this product and it has other uses as well. Another original Dick Quinn formula, Health Food Caps contain Alfalfa, Garlic, Gotu Kola, Cayenne, Kelp, Onion, Ginger and Lecithin. Alfalfa and Kelp are extremely nourishing herbs which reportedly even protect you from the hazards of radiation. They also help cleanse the body. Gotu Kola is a great circulatory system herb, an anti-aging herb which boosts mental energy and alleviates depression. All the herbs together make a great skin formula and can also enhance the immune system. I like this one.

Cayenne Thinking Caps: This original Dick Quinn formula contains Gotu Kola, Cayenne, Gingko Biloba, Peppermint and Lecithin. This one is good for people of all ages, anyone who could use a little more energy and mental clarity¡and who couldn't use that? I give it to my children to help them get the most out of their day. My daughter Heather uses it for energy and to promote clear skin. So far this year, she's an A student. Last year, without Thinking Caps, she was a C student. Although the credit goes entirely to Heather for working so hard, I think the Thinking Caps help give her the energy she needs to do what she needs to do.

"C's" The Day Caps: This is one of the newest additions to the Heartfoods line. It contains Vitamin C, Echinacea, Cayenne and Ginger. Product literature recommends it for daily use and calls it "sunshine in a bottle." Cute, but I wouldn't recommend this for every day. Echinacea, a natural anti-biotic, should not be taken on a daily basis unless some evidence of infection is present. I use this when one of my kids is sickịthe patient gets it, and the rest of us will take it for a week or so, just to ensure we don't catch whatever the patient has. So far, so good. But for daily use, better to use Heart Food Caps or Thinking Caps.

Hawthorn Plus! Caps: Do not contain Cayenne, but do contain Hawthorn Berries, Garlic, Heartwort and Onion. Another newer product, this would be good to take if you have a heart condition but are unable to take Cayenne. Most people can take Cayenne and it's worth looking for a product that's comfortable for you containing Cayenne. The Heart Food Caps for example, would provide many more benefits. But if someone won't take Cayenne, try this.

Cayenne Stress Food Caps: Originally called "Happy Caps," this Dick Quinn formula contains Catnip, Valerian, Peppermint, Cayenne, Ginger and Lecithin. This is a good product to try if life is stressing you out, as it gives energy and relaxes you at the same time. Catnip, Peppermint and Ginger settle nervous stomachs and are soothing, calming herbs. Valerian alleviates stress, is a great sleep aid, regulates the heartbeat and is a muscle relaxant. Try this if you have a tension-headache or sore back. You'll be amazed at the difference.

Nite Time Caps: Were originally "Night Caps," but only the name has been changed of this Dick Quinn formula. Containing Valerian, Passion Flower, Skullcap, Peppermint and Lecithin, Nite Time Caps are the best sleep-aid I've ever tried. We give it to the kids to ensure a restful nights sleep. All the herbs are anti-stress and relaxation herbs. A wonderful product.

Every Day: Contains Licorice, Kelp, Yellow Dock and Heartwort. A Dick Quinn formula, this is promoted as a women's product, but men could see benefits, too. Licorice is a very nutritive herb, is good for the liver and feeds the adrenal glands. Yellow Dock is a blood cleanser.

Women's Day: Is a Dick Quinn formula that I take every day. It contains Crampbark, Dong Quai, Peppermint and Dandelion. This is a good product to ease the troubles of PMS or menstruation. Crampbark stops cramps, Dong Quai is a major women's herb, easing stress and regulating cycles. Peppermint soothes and calms the body and mind. Dandelion fights fluid retention. An excellent product.

Afterglow: Is another Dick Quinn formula I take every day. It contains: Passion Flower, Dong Quai, Damiana, Hawthorn Berries, Kelp and Sarsaparilla. Promoted as a product for those going through menopause, this can be taken by any female. Passion Flower relieves stress, Sarsaparilla feeds the adrenals and provides energy. Damiana is the woman's sex herb and is used for a wide variety of menstrual complaints.

Cayenne Keep It Up Caps: An original Dick Quinn formula, I hate to say it, but I don't take this one. A good product as far as maintaining sexual health and potency, it contains Saw Palmetto, Damiana, Licorice, Sarsaparilla and Cayenne. All the herbs feed the adrenals and Saw Palmetto prevents and treats prostate problems. I don't take this one, because I prefer a formula also containing Siberian Ginseng.

Heartfoods also has a line of natural insect repellants: **Tickweed Plus** and **Citronella Plus.** The Tickweed product is supposed to repel ticks, the Citronella product flies and mosquitos I've used the Citronella product with some success, the Tickweed one with less success. They smell great though and work on people of any age and animals, too.

Remember, these products are only a few of the many herbal products on the market. Take some time to compare prices and formula before you buy. You may be able to find a product that is similar but much less expensive.

Dear Reader,

Whenever I can, I get water from the well over at Lake Harriet in Minneapolis. I love the way it tastes and never seems to go flat. Al Watson says it's full of bacteria, but I don't let that spoil it for me. These are friendly bugs; they like me. They even taste good.

I met a tall, dignified man at the well a few weeks ago. I don't know how old he was—65 maybe. His eyes were sunken behind dark rings. He seemed weak and unsteady, so I urged him to let me pump the water for him, but he insisted on pumping some of it himself. It was important to him to show me he could do it. He wasn't an invalid. His self esteem wouldn't permit it.

"My doctor told me to get some exercise," he explained weakly. "It's this damned chemotherapy," he shrugged with disgust, tears in his eyes. "It's terrible. Terrible." He seemed to recoil at the memory of the pain and sickness. He couldn't look at me when he spoke of it. "It cost $85,000.

I remembered the studies I'd read. How they performed autopsies on cancer patients and found they hadn't died of cancer, the chemotherapy killed them. They were murdered, treated to death. "Tortured to death," as one poor soul said in a newspaper story I read. "Please don't let them torture me to death," he had begged his son. They did it anyway. He reminded me of this old man at the well.

The man at the well didn't even have cancer. His doctor gave him chemotherapy to prevent the "possible" onset of adult leukemia. He was a "good candidate" because of his age and insurance. He suffered untold agony from "preventive treatment" that nearly killed him. He wasn't sick; they made him sick. They tortured him for the $85,000. His doctor got his fee; used car salesmen call it a commission, but they're more honest. The price is never too high when someone else pays.

"My kids want me to go to the Mexican clinics next time, but I don't know," he said. "I wouldn't want my doctor to find out.

He's a young intern and he's just about to be named an associate. I don't want to do anything that might get in the way of that."

The poor, dear man. Barely emerging from the nightmare alive, yet more concerned about his doctor's career than his own anguish. The angel of death profits from an old man's pain, exploits his decency and betrays his trust. A kind, valued, caring human being is tortured to serve arrogance and greed.

We must be protected from people like that old man's doctor. We are all patients some time in our lives. We must help each other to health. That's why we started our newsletter.

<u>Help Yourself to Health</u> explains your health care options honestly. We don't profit from your illness—we're here to help you help yourself.

Good health to you!

Dick Quinn

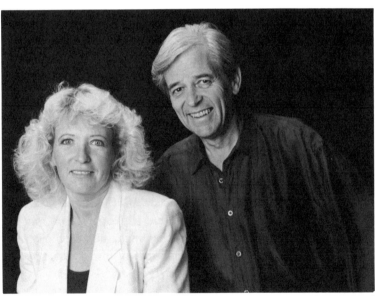

Dick and his daughter Kelly learned herbalism through practical experience.

chamomile: 25, 26, 55, 82, 92, 99, 109, 130
chaparral: 9, 14, 92, 103
chaste tree (vitex): 107
chemotherapy: 7
cherries: 48
chickweed: 30, 48, 79, 92, 127
childbirth: 108
cholesterol: 1, 13, 15, 113
chromium picolinate: 79
chronic fatigue syndrome: 104
cleavers: 8-9
cloves: 6, 14
coffee: 3, 66
comfrey: 25, 37, 91, 106, 110, 115
common cold: 112
congestion: 2, 3
contraceptives: 74, 81
cornsilk: 45, 105, 122
cosmetics: 31-32
cough: 112, 167
crampbark: 112, 114, 116

damiana: 106, 125, 127
dandelion: 109, 113, 122, 138-140
dandruff: 35, 82
decoction: 60
dehydration: 11, 79
depression: 27, 96, 105, 106
devil's claw: 141
diarrhea: 2, 51, 54, 81
distilled water: 40
dong quai: 7, 107
dragon cocktail: 20, 50, 168

earache/swimmer's ear: 11
echinacea (echinacea augusti-folia): 8-9, 57, 92, 115, 127, 137, 138

ephedra: 3, 112
essential oils: 97-100
estrogen replacement therapy: 107
eucalyptus oil: 99
evening primrose oil: 144
exercise: 5, 66, 72, 76, 78
eyebright: 72

false unicorn root: 72, 107, 121, 140
fatigue/weakness: 139
fats: 15-20
female problems: 45, 56-58, 100-110
fennel: 55, 99, 121, 129, 140
fenugreek: 120, 130
feverfew: 71, 102, 143
flu: 46, 54

garlic: 50, 57, 66, 102, 104, 121, 124, 127, 129, 130, 137, 138, 140, 141, 167
gas/stomach aches: 46, 53-56
germanium: 99, 107
ginger: 11, 22, 54, 73, 99, 122, 130, 138, 139, 140-141
ginko biloba: 73, 128, 139, 143
goldenseal: 3, 8-9, 51, 92, 106, 130, 137, 138, 140
gotu kola: 65, 73, 124, 127-128, 139, 167, 169-170
gout: 47
guggalo: 79

hair: 11, 22-26
hair dye recipes: 38
hair dyes: 37
hair rinses: 25-36, 37
hair sprays: 24
Halcion: 5, 63

hawthorn: 138, 179
hayfever: 46
headaches/migraines: 11, 69-75, 136
heart disease: 46
heat units (h.u.): 21-22
herbal formulas: 149-155, 161-165, 173, 174, 178, 179-182
hismanal: 2, 70
homeopathy: 1, 85-89
hops: 6, 72, 103, 146
horseradish: 55, 92
horsetail: 92

immune system: 2-4, 104-105
indigestion: 53-56
infection: 51, 56-58, 136-138
infusion: 60-63
insomnia: 4-6

jellyfish: 12
juniper berries: 99, 139, 140

kelp: 40, 45, 122
kidneys: 13, 45, 105

lady's slipper: 107
lavender: 99
laxative: 171-173
lead poisoning: 40-41
lecithin: 107
licorice: 15, 82, 139
liver: 26-30, 83
lobelia: 3, 82, 122, 130, 138, 146
lymphatic system: 7-10, 12

marigold: 25, 57
marshmallow root: 105, 121, 140
menopause: 107-108

menstruation: 74, 109
mistletoe: 107, 122, 143
motherwort: 109
myrrh: 8-9, 99, 106, 137, 138, 141

nausea: 11, 51, 53-56, 136
nettles: 26, 45, 105, 109, 110
neem: 15
nutmeg: 99

oats: 55
oatseed: 82
onion: 40, 50, 124, 129
Oregon grape root: 140, 141
osteoporosis: 81, 109

parsley: 45, 105, 109, 138, 139, 140
passion flower: 6, 67
pau d'arco: 57, 103, 137
peach bark: 92
pennyroyal: 99, 109, 122
peppermint: 2, 51, 55, 82, 99, 122, 129
pest control: 10, 11, 41-44
pesticides: 41-44
plantain: 79, 92
PMS: 74, 109, 118
prostate: 44-45
pumpkin seeds: 45, 140, 142

radiation: 160
recipes: 18-19, 30, 48
red clover: 14, 25, 106
red raspberry: 51, 54, 107, 109, 122, 130, 141, 142
Rogaine: 38, 39
rose hips: 72, 122, 141
rosemary: 25, 37, 62, 72, 98-99, 119, 147

Magazines and Periodicals:

British Medical Journal
Cancer Facts and Figures from the American Cancer Society
International Journal of Cancer
Journal of the American Medical Association
New England Journal of Medicine
The New York Times
Newsweek
Parapalegia
Psychosomatics
Whittaker Wellness Letter

Books:

Health Through God's Pharmacy by Maria Treben

The Complete Medicinal Herbal by Penelope Ody

Prescription for Natural Healing by James F. Balch, M.D. and Phyllis A. Balch, C.N.C.

The Magic of Nature's Healing Herbs from Globe Communications Corporation

Natural Health Remedies from Globe Communications Corporation

Health Handbook by Louise Tenney

Pocket Reference Book by Debra Nuzzi

A Beginner's Guide to Homeopathy from Medicine From Nature

Left for Dead by Dick Quinn with Shannon Quinn and Colin Quinn

The Male Herbal by James Green

The Herbal for Mother and Child by Anne McIntyre

Rodale's Illustrated Encyclopedia of Herbs from Rodale

Reducing the Risk of Alzheimer's by Dr. Michael Weiner

The Book of Herbs by Edmond Bordeaux Sze'kely

Scientific Validation of Herbal Medicine by Daniel B. Mowry

Family Herbal by Peter and Barbara Theiss

Fighting Infections With Herbs/Sexually Transmitted Infections by Linda Rector-Page N.D., Ph.D.

Encyclopedia of Fruits, Vegetables and Herbs by John Heinerman

Back to Eden by Jethro Kloss

Mastering Herbalism by Paul Huson

Herbs for Healthful Living by Richard Lucas

The Healing Power of Herbs by May Bethel

Historical Dictionary

Bull Cookbook by Leonard Herter

Vitamin C and the Common Cold and Flu by Linus Pauling

How to Live Longer and Feel Better by Linus Pauling

Herbally Yours by Penny C. Royal

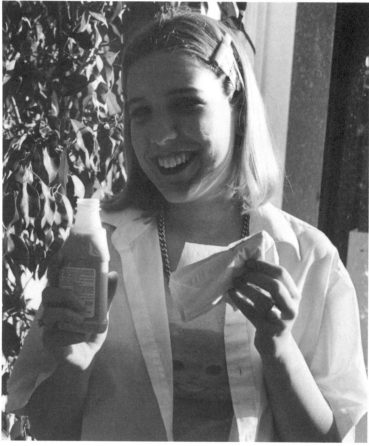

Shannon keeps her complexion clear with facials using a common diarrhea remedy.

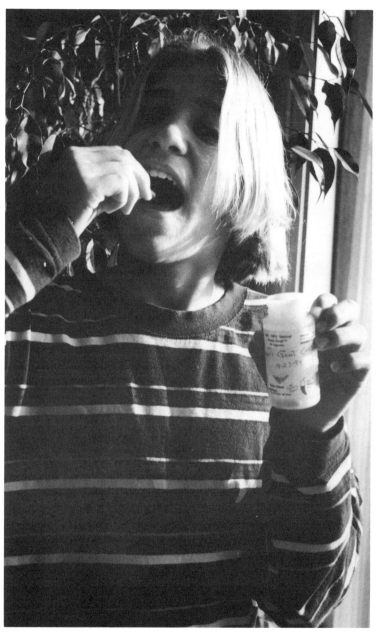

Kelly's son Quinn discovered he had gout at the ripe old age of 10. The solution: Queen of the Meadow herb."

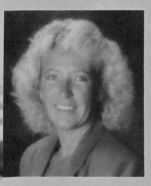

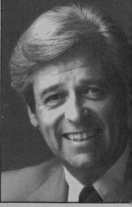
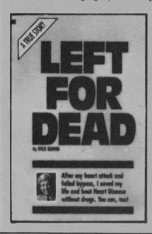